19.95

QV748'

Fundamentals
of Primary Care
Prescribing

LI............CES

S...............TAL

Fundamentals of Primary Care Prescribing

Edited by Brian Crichton
BSc (Hons) MBChB FRCGP Cert. DC

Royal College of General Practitioners
London · 2006

LEARNING RESOURCES
CENTRE
SHELTON HOSPITAL

The Royal College of General Practitioners was founded in 1952 with this object:

"To encourage, foster and maintain the highest possible standards in general practice and for that purpose to take or join with others in taking steps consistent with the charitable nature of that object which may assist towards the same."

Among its responsibilities under its Royal Charter the College is entitled to:

"Diffuse information on all matters affecting general practice and issue such publications as may assist the object of the College."

British Library Cataloguing-in-Publication Data
A catalogue record for this book is available from the British Library

© Royal College of General Practitioners, 2006
Published by the Royal College of General Practitioners, 2006
14 Princes Gate, Hyde Park, London SW7 1PU

All rights reserved. No part of this publication may be reproduced, stored in a retrieval system, or transmitted, in any form or by any means, electronic, mechanical, photocopying, recording or otherwise without the prior permission of the Royal College of General Practitioners.

Disclaimer
This publication is intended for the use of medical practitioners in the UK and not for patients. The authors, editors and publisher have taken care to ensure that the information contained in this book is correct to the best of their knowledge, at the time of publication. Whilst efforts have been made to ensure the accuracy of the information presented, particularly that related to the prescription of drugs, the authors, editors and publisher cannot accept liability for information that is subsequently shown to be wrong. Readers are advised to check that the information, especially that related to drug usage, complies with information contained in the *British National Formulary*, or equivalent, or manufacturers' datasheets, and that it complies with the latest legislation and standards of practice.

Designed and typeset by Robert Updegraff
Printed by Latimer Trend
Indexed by Carol Ball
ISBN: 0 85084 305 7

Contents

Foreword

A good general practice consultation is a complex event. It involves a wide range of skills and tasks, one of the most important of which is prescribing. General practitioners have often been criticised for being too quick on the draw with their prescription pads, although this is heard less often today. When used responsibly, the prescription is the most common effective action a prescriber can take.

Given the vast numbers of prescriptions issued every day, it is not surprising that some are incorrect and a very few frankly damaging to the patient. Unfortunately, some adverse reactions and effects are unavoidable – but many are avoidable. Beyond straight safety issues lie questions of appropriateness, cost-effectiveness, innovation, guidelines and the creation of medical dependency.

Technology can help. When allergies, contraindications or adverse reactions have been entered, computerised decision support can offer protection against prescribing inappropriately. Ready access to information can help the prescriber be better informed on medicines and devices, including guidelines and policies. Computer-generated pathways of care can coordinate care for patients with complex needs. Despite all of this support, the prescribing decision will largely remain one of clinical judgement within clear policies that encourage safety.

Since prescribing is such an important topic for doctors, nurses, pharmacists and patients, it is good to find a level-headed book reviewing the area. In these pages lies a wealth of wisdom that should be noted well by young – and not so young – doctors, nurses and pharmacists prescribing in primary care.

Professor Mike Pringle
University of Nottingham
March 2006

Preface

This book is mainly intended for prospective prescribers in primary care, although final-year medical students and GP registrars will also find it useful. It aims to provide a broad consideration of the disciplines involved in prescribing, and interested readers are directed towards the relevant references for further reading.

Prescribing occupies a central role in management of our patients. It is at its most effective as part of a patient-centred approach to the consultation and equips us with a vehicle to help relieve both real and potential suffering.

The pace of change with the development of new drugs and the increasing degree of chronic disease management in primary care stretches prescribers to the full. Despite these challenges the rewards are high for both prescribers and patients alike.

It is my hope that readers will find this book useful as an aid to laying down the fundamentals necessary for good and effective prescribing.

Brian Crichton
2006

Acknowledgements

I would like to take this opportunity to express my gratitude to some special people who have provided help and advice during the development of this publication: Dr Rodger Charlton, Senior Lecturer at the Department of General Practice, Warwick University Medical School; Professor Donald Singer, Professor of Pharmacology, University of Warwick Medical School; Mr Mark Greener, medical writing adviser; Mrs Tho Lam, Community Pharmacist, Solihull; and Mrs Fiona Beadle, Hospital and Practice Support Pharmacist, Solihull Primary Care Trust.

Finally, I would like to thank the Royal College of General Practitioners for its help and support in the publication of this work.

Abbreviations

ABPI	Association of the British Pharmaceutical Industry
ACBS	Advisory Committee on Borderline Substances
ACE	angiotensin-converting enzyme
ADRs	adverse drug reactions
BMA	British Medical Association
BNF	*British National Formulary*
CBA	cost–benefit analysis
CD	controlled drugs
CEA	cost-effectiveness analysis
CHD	coronary heart disease
CMA	cost minimisation analysis
CNS	central nervous system
CPD	continuing professional development
CSM	Committee on Safety of Medicines
CUA	cost utility analysis
CYP	cytochrome P450
DCFS	NHS Counter Fraud Service
DMARDs	disease-modifying antirheumatic drugs
DoH	Department of Health
DSRU	Drug Safety Research Unit
EMEA	European Medicine Evaluation Agency
FBC	full blood count
GABA$_A$	gamma-aminobutyric acid type A
GCP	good clinical practice
GMC	General Medical Council
GMS	General Medical Services
HGP	Human Genome Project
HRT	hormone replacement therapy
INR	International Normalised Ratio
IP	independent prescriber
MCA	Medicines Control Agency
MHRA	Medicines and Healthcare products Regulatory Agency
MIMS	*Monthly Index of Medical Specialities*
MPS	Medical Protection Society
NICE	National Institute for Health and Clinical Excellence
NMC	Nursing and Midwifery Council
NNT	number needed to treat
NPSA	National Patient Safety Agency
NPT	near patient testing

NSAIDs	non-steroidal anti-inflammatory drugs
NSFs	National Service Frameworks
NTIS	National Teratology Information Service
NVQ	National Vocational Qualification
OCP	oral contraceptive pill
OTC	over-the-counter medicines
PACT	Prescribing Analysis and Cost
PCOs	primary care organisations
PCT	Primary Care Trust
PDRM	preventable drug-related morbidity
PEM	prescription-event monitoring
PMDs	Prescribing Monitoring Documents
POM	prescription-only medicine
PPA	Prescription Pricing Authority
PPARs	peroxisome proliferator-activated receptors
PUs	prescribing units
QALY	Quality Adjusted Life Year
R&D	research and development
RPSGB	Royal Pharmaceutical Society of Great Britain
SAMM	safety assessment of marketed medicines
SLS	Selected List Scheme
SOPs	standard operating procedures
SP	supplementary prescriber
TB	tuberculosis
TFTs	thyroid function tests
TNF	tumour necrosis factor
UKCC	United Kingdom Central Council for Nurses, Midwives and Health Visitors
WHO	World Health Organization

Contributors

Professor Tony Avery is a GP in Nottingham and Head of the Division of Primary Care at the University of Nottingham. He has longstanding research interests in prescribing and patient safety in primary care. He is a member of the Joint Formulary Committee of the *British National Formulary*, Consultant Editor of the journal *Prescriber* and a member of the Expert Prioritisation Panel of the National Patient Safety Agency.

Fiona Beadle MPharm has worked as a clinical pharmacist in a hospital and a community pharmacy, as well as at the Committee on Safety of Medicines West Midlands Adverse Drug Reaction unit. She is a member of a hospital medicines safety committee and has been on the drug and therapeutics committee involved with the managed introduction of new drugs. Since 1995 she has been a practice support pharmacist with Solihull Primary Care Trust, working with GPs and other members of the practice healthcare team to support the development and application of high-quality, safe, cost-effective, rational and evidence-based prescribing.

Professor Colin Bradley MD MICGP was appointed as the Foundation Professor of General Practice at University College Cork in 1997. He was previously a senior lecturer at the University of Birmingham and a lecturer at the University of Manchester. He has a particular research interest in the prescribing behaviour of general practitioners. His doctoral work was on decisions GPs make about whether or not to prescribe. He has also conducted work on how GPs and specialists introduce new drugs into their clinical practices and on patients' attitudes to over-the-counter medicines. He was a member of the Benzodiazepine Committee that reported to the Minister of Health and Children in 2002.

Dr Brian Crichton BSc (Hons) MBChB FRCGP Cert. DC has degrees in biochemistry and chemistry as well as medicine, and became a GP principal in 1993. In 1996 he became a GP trainer and, in 2002, an undergraduate teacher in the Department of General Practice at Warwick University Medical School, where he is now an honorary senior lecturer. He is one of the prescribing advisers to the RCGP and has publications in many different areas of prescribing. Further to this he is a passionate GP educationalist and has lectured locally, nationally and internationally on therapeutics and prescribing issues.

Dr Gerard Panting MA MB BS FFFLM FRCGP DMJ spent 12 years in the NHS before moving to the Medical Protection Society (MPS) in 1987, initially as a medico-legal adviser, then as Head of UK Medical Services and latterly as Director of Communications and Policy. He left in 2006 to pursue a number of other interests, but continues to advise MPS on policy and risk management. He has enormous experience in designing and delivering educational programmes, and is well known as a presenter, writer and specialist commentator in the UK and overseas.

Professor Tom Walley MBBCh MD FRCP FRCPI MRCGP qualified in Dublin in 1980. He was appointed consultant physician in the Royal Liverpool University Hospital in 1991 and Professor of Clinical Pharmacology in 1994. His research interests are in pharmacoepidemiology, pharmacoeconomics and undergraduate and postgraduate teaching to improve prescribing. He has published over 200 articles in peer-reviewed journals. In 2003, he was appointed director of the national Health Technology Assessment Programme, and director of the UK infrastructure for reviews, responsible for the promotion and management of the Cochrane groups in the UK.

A brief history of prescribing

Brian Crichton

Since the dawn of time, witch doctors, wise women and other healers have collected and formulated biologically active chemicals to cure or prevent disease and injury. As Jackson notes,[1] the knowledge that plants, minerals and animal products can heal is probably as old as the human race. The Canadian-born, Oxford University Professor of Medicine Sir William Osler commented that the desire to take medicines is one of those features that sets hominids apart from other animals.[2] Not surprisingly, traditional medicines often had considerable social, intellectual, economic and cultural value.[3]

So, in one way or another, prescribing and prescribers have been important parts of human culture for millennia. Indeed, testament to this long history is borne each time a prescription is made. The ancient Egyptians used the eye of Horus to describe fractions and the proportion of each ingredient in a medicine. Horus was the son of two of the main gods in Egyptian mythology, Isis and Osiris. Horus had an evil uncle (Seth) who murdered Osiris. Horus then did battle with Seth to avenge his father's murder. During the fight, Seth plucked out Horus's left eye and tore it apart. Thoth (the god of wisdom and magic) found the eye, pieced it together and added some magic. He returned the eye to Horus, who in turn gave it to his murdered father Osiris, thereby bringing him back to life. The 'Rx' symbol is a direct descendant of this dissection of the eye of Horus. Incidentally, the ancient Egyptian healers were also the first to write prescriptions.[4]

For millennia, medicine often relied on sympathetic magic – the idea that like cures like. An ancient Egyptian headache remedy, for example, involved heating catfish skull until it turned to ashes and then boiling with oil. The sufferer rubbed the oil into his or her head for four days.[5] That isn't to say that the traditional medicines weren't valuable; many herbs are biologically active. And the placebo effect – augmented by the ritual of magic – was potent. Today, of course, prescribing is based on scientific principles, rather than magic. But the art of medicine remains important for prescribers, when, for example, developing a therapeutic relationship with patients.

The classical period

From all the healing traditions that emerged over the years, classical writers cast the longest shadow over prescribers and prescribing. Greeks in the fifth century BC could call on healers from several medical schools, including the Aesculapian, Cnidian and Hippocratic schools. The Hippocratic tradition, of course, emerged pre-eminent.[6,7,8]

Founded on the island of Cos around 430 BC, the Hippocratic tradition viewed the problems from the physician's perspective. This set the Cos physicians apart from the rest of the medical schools. So, for instance, one volume of Hippocratic writing called the *Prognosis* – a term still used today – used past knowledge combined with current observation to determine future outcomes. Furthermore, Hippocratic doctors emphasised the importance of basing treatment around the patient and observing the benefits of the treatment in practice. That's still a valid rule for prescribers even in this post-genomic era. Indeed, the *Corpus Hippocraticum* – the group's collection of 58 documents, which were certainly not all written by Hippocrates – still has the potential to offer insights into a disease. Of course, many doctors still swear the Hippocratic oath, which codifies some central principles for prescribers today.

As Greek civilisation began to decline, the Roman Empire increased in importance. Nevertheless, Roman healers still followed the path mapped out in Cos, although they augmented the *Corpus* with observations of their own. For example, the blood sports in the arena contributed to the Romans' knowledge of anatomy, although on one occasion when physicians gathered to witness the dissection of an elephant, imperial cooks took the heart![9]

The Roman physician Galen (AD 129–200) is the most prominent of these classical scholars. Galen remained an influential figure for an amazing 15 centuries and some of the principles he pioneered remain valid even today. Galen, for example, seems to have been among the first physicians to insist on the purity of medicines.[1] However, Galen's pervasive influence was not always benevolent. For example, his suggestion that blood ebbed and flowed hindered the widespread acceptance of Harvey's theory of blood circulation.[10] Also, Galen believed that pus was an essential part of healing. Many thousands of people probably died from infections because of this mistaken belief.[2]

These historical examples show that prescribers should never take so-called authoritative texts at face value. Medicine advances rapidly. So prescribers should always endeavour, as far as possible, to remain 'on top' of the literature that impacts on their practice.

The Arabic period

After the Roman Empire declined and fell, the Islamic world became the centre of medical learning. During the ninth century, Arabic scholars translated many Greek medical books, which they again augmented from experience. This laid the foundation for Arabic scholars' considerable understanding of pharmacognosy, pharmacology and prescribing more generally. For example, Arabs developed pharmacy as an independent discipline from medicine, pre-dating the distinction in the West by several centuries. Overall, Arabic physicians and scientists gradually produced a considerable body of rational, empirical, systematic knowledge about the effectiveness of medicinal plants and drugs.[11]

During this translation and assimilation, Arabic scholars also adopted a technique that is still widely used in modern medical literature: the case history.[12] For example, rare side effects and drug–drug interactions are often first reported in case histories.

Islamic medicine's golden age stretched from the ninth to the eleventh centuries, which was a period of rapid development across art, literature and science. For example, the surgeon Abdul Qassim Al-Zahrawi wrote the 30-volume *Kitab Al Tasrif Liman Ajiza* and *Al-Talif*, an encyclopaedia encapsulating the state of medical and surgical knowledge in the tenth-century Hijarah.[13] Avicenna's *Canon of Medicine*, translated from Arabic into Latin by Gerard of Cremona, represented the 'supreme authority' across the Christian and Islamic world for around 600 years.[14]

During the eleventh century, Christian doctors began to recover classical texts from Muslim and Jewish physicians, especially in Byzantine Spain and Arabian Africa.[15] By the twelfth century, scholars in Italy and Spain had translated most of the augmented Arabic texts into Latin.[11] These translated textbooks were used in the growing number of medical schools, such as Montpellier in southern France. From the fifteenth century, scholars added Greek manuscripts to the Latin texts.[16]

The Enlightenment

The next turning point in the history of prescribing came during the Enlightenment. The Aristotelian, Neo-Platonic and Hermetic philosophies that dominated science during the Renaissance fell under the onslaught of a Newtonian vision of a universe governed by mathematical laws. This mechanistic vision inevitably influenced biology. One paradigm viewed the human body as 'a system of pulleys, springs and levers, pipes and vessels'. The laws of hydraulics governed the flow of fluids in the body.

Physicians also challenged the classical view of medicine, in part from economic self-interest. The Hippocratic tradition emphasised nature's innate healing ability; physicians and their prescriptions acted only as nature's handmaidens. However, the medical profession was becoming increasingly professional, and to protect their elite professional status, doctors became increasingly protectionist. As a result, physicians set themselves up as 'experts' in disease management. While paying lip service to the Hippocratic tradition, physicians suggested that the body's innate ability sufficed to heal only the most trivial conditions. In all other cases, nature needed professional help.

Meanwhile, consumerism began to spread through the social strata. So during the Enlightenment people from relatively economically deprived classes also expected to receive effective prescriptions. This demand helped fuel the rise of apothecaries, chemists and druggists to meet the needs of the poorer segments of the population. In the seventeenth century, apothecaries in England were part of the Grocers' Company. But a growing raft of specific regulations as well as commercial and professional pressures led to a split and the foundation of the Society of Apothecaries in 1618. Members of the Society of Apothecaries won a key legal suit (known as the Rose Case) against the Royal College of Physicians in the House of Lords in 1704, which ruled that apothecaries could both prescribe and dispense medicines. This led directly to the evolution of the apothecary into the first general practitioners, offering advice to patients who could not afford to consult a doctor.

The same year as the apothecaries founded their society, the *London Pharmacopoeia* was published. Following the formulations in the *London Pharmacopoeia* was mandatory for doctors, apothecaries and others preparing prescriptions. The *London Pharmacopoeia* was the first national pharmacopoeia. However, pharmacopoeia had appeared before, in the German version published in 1546.

The idea that disease could be treated by prescribing chemicals rather than herbs – which began with the Swiss physician Paracelsus (see Chapter 2) – began to become increasingly influential. For example, Thomas Beddos predicted in 1793 that chemistry would lead to a safe and efficacious remedy for tuberculosis. Ultimately, his prediction proved right – but it took several centuries to reach fruition. The *Pharmacopoeia* reflected the increasingly scientific attitude that characterised the spirit of the age. Viper flesh, pike jaw and unicorn horn all disappeared during the Enlightenment.

During the nineteenth century, general practitioners split from the chemists. The Apothecaries Act introduced compulsory apprenticeship and formal qualification. The licentiateship became the commonest qualification among general practitioners. However, by 1840 only about a third of those practising medicine qualified by examination.

Chemists – as their name suggests – dealt in chemicals. Once they split from the apothecaries, chemists merged with druggists, who dealt in animal and vegetable products. In 1815, an act of parliament legally established that chemists and druggists could by right purchase, compound, dispense and sell drugs.[17] It is from this group that our community pharmacists emerged.

Against this background, the nineteenth-century physicians increasingly saw themselves as gentlemen practising the 'noble art' of medicine. Physicians regarded surgeons and apothecaries as closer to tradesmen than gentlemen. As a result, the physicians tried to distance themselves from anything that smacked of manual labour including bleeding, purging and prescribing.

This trend culminated in 1844, when the Royal College of Surgeons of England instigated a new charter that created a small number of Fellows. After this time, Fellowship of the College could be achieved by examination only. However, most of the College's members were general practitioners and, as a result of the charter, became disenfranchised. So, in December of the same year, the National Association of General Practitioners in Medicine, Surgery and Midwifery was founded.

The need for more effective regulation of the growing number of physicians and prescribers soon became apparent. In 1847, a Parliamentary Select Committee made a number of recommendations about the registration and practice of medicine and surgery. The 1858 Medical Act established the General Council of Medical Education and Registration (General Medical Council). Today, medical practitioners must register with the Council, which supervises training and handles serious disciplinary issues including those surrounding mis-prescribing.

During this period, pharmacists were isolating the active ingredients from numerous herbal remedies. They isolated, for example, morphine from the opium poppy in 1806, quinine from cinchona bark in 1820, nicotine from the tobacco plant in 1828 and atropine from the deadly nightshade in 1883. These isolates proved economically lucrative. In 1885, for instance, Merck sold over 80,000 kilograms of cocaine. The isolates allowed researchers to gain some insight into the mode of action of chemicals. Nicotine, for example, stimulates receptors on neuromuscular junctions and ganglia. This is reflected in their name: nicotinic receptors. Atropine blocks the action of acetylcholine. These discoveries laid the intellectual foundation for modern prescribing.

The advances in drugs did not just emerge from studies of natural remedies. Carbonisation of hard coal powered nineteenth-century industry and society more widely. Coal gas and coke fuelled civic lighting and the industrial furnaces respectively. However, carbonisation left behind a huge amount of coal tar. Fortunately, chemists found that, with simple modifications, this mix of chemicals could yield almost any colour in the spectrum. The English chemist Sir William Henry Perkin made the first so-called aniline dye in 1856 while attempting to synthesise quinine.[18] Aniline dyes formed the chemical basis of several drugs including the phenothiazines, such as the major tranquillisers promethazine and chlorpromazine, the first neuroleptic that transformed the management of schizophrenia.

A young student working at the University of Strasbourg between 1872 and 1874 noted that these dyes bound selectively to different tissues. The student, Paul Ehrlich, developed the idea that parasites, micro-organisms and cancer cells expressed different 'chemo receptors' from other tissues. So chemists should be able to exploit these differences therapeutically[19] and develop 'magic bullets' targeted to the specific tissue or organism. Then, in 1905, J.N. Langley characterised receptors as switches. Langley suggested that antagonists block the receptor, thereby turning it off. Agonists do the opposite. The idea of receptors, together with the increasing diversity of chemicals, forms the basis of the modern pharmaceutical industry.

Until the early years of the twentieth century, medicine was practised predominately in hospitals or, if it could be afforded, by doctors visiting the patient's home. A few medical philanthropists staffed charity hospitals. Clearly, this system did not meet the public health need – as the overflowing wards in the workhouses proved. So in 1920 the Dawson report suggested establishing primary health centres in the community. During the Second World War, the UK established the Emergency Bed Service to care for the injured. And, in 1942, an inter-departmental committee led by Sir William Beveridge identified health care as a basic principle for a viable social security.

Meanwhile, pharmacological advances continued apace – exemplified by the antibiotic miracle. In the late nineteenth century, researchers recognised that certain synthetic azo dyes eradicated some bacteria in the test tube. Paul Ehrlich discovered, around 1909–10, arsphenamine – a drug derived from arsenic – that proved to be the first clinically effective syphilis treatment that did not have serious, dose-limiting side effects. Over the next few years, numerous other chemical antibiotics followed including the sulphonamides – originally derived from a red dye called prontosil rubrum.

However, infections still killed thousands. Tuberculosis, for example, was the white plague. The answer came from an unexpected source: a mould. Ironically, researchers noted the mould's antibacterial properties as long ago as 1875. But it was not until Alexander Fleming famously left a petri dish of bacteria open (1928), when he went on holiday, which became colonised with the pencillium mould, that the antibiotic era dawned.

Nevertheless, it was still several years – 1938 – before penicillin's commercialisation was begun by E. Chain, Howard Florey and their collaborators.[19] Drug companies began mass-producing penicillin in 1943. However, penicillin resistance was first reported in 1947.[20] Although penicillin was followed by erythromycin, tetracyclines, macrolides, cephalosporins and so on, bacterial resistance remains a serious problem even today. To help combat this, several antibiotics with novel modes of action are in development, which may help prescribers stay one step ahead of bacterial evolution.

Over the course of the years covered in this chapter, prescribing moved from plant-based therapies to high-tech medicines aimed at a particular molecular target – a principle best exemplified by aspirin and the other non-steroidal anti-inflammatory drugs (NSAIDs). Traditional healers used plants containing salicylates to treat inflammation and alleviate pain for millennia. But the modern story opens in 1763 when the Reverend Edward Stone of Chipping Norton in Oxfordshire reported to the Royal Society that a dram of dried willow bark in tea, small beer or water cured fever in most of the 50 people who tried it.[21]

In 1829, the French chemist Pierre Leroux isolated salicin from willow bark and showed that it reduced fever. Over the next few years, chemical manipulations led to sodium salicylate and acetylsalicylic acid. Felix Hoffman, a chemist working for the German company Bayer, showed that acetylsalicylic acid alleviated the inflammation endured by his arthritic father. Acetylsalicylic acid was launched as aspirin in 1899. The drug gained a new lease of life when it emerged as effective in the primary and secondary treatment of cardiovascular disease.[22] Aspirin was grouped into the class of drugs called NSAIDs. This group grew in number, with all reducing pain and inflammation, but also unfortunately increasing the risk of gastrointestinal erosions, ulcers and bleeds, which can prove fatal. Doctors can now prescribe, due to an evolution in NSAID development, COX-2 selective inhibitors for higher-risk patients as these are thought not to cause the serious gastrointestinal side effects caused by other NSAIDs. However, COX-2 selective inhibitors remain effective anti-inflammatory drugs.

Over the same years, these dramatic advances in pharmacological sciences were matched by equally notable social changes. For example, the 1944 white paper *National Health Service*[23] established, for the first time, the principle that 'everybody, irrespective of means, age, sex or occupation shall have equal opportunity to benefit from the best and most up-to-date medical and allied services available'. The white paper added that services should be 'comprehensive and free of charge and should promote good health as well as treating sickness and disease'.

The white paper reflected a consensus that emerged about the need for social security in the wake of the Second World War. This led to the foundation of the NHS in 1948. In the new NHS, GPs became responsible for personal medical care and acted as gatekeepers for hospital access, specialist care and sickness benefit. The GP's growing importance led to the Royal Society of Medicine forming a General Practice section in 1950. Two years later, on 19 November 1952, the College of General Practitioners (later the Royal College of General Practitioners, RCGP) was founded.

Since then, the NHS has undergone numerous changes – including the introduction of the internal market, fund holding, primary care organisations, league tables, the National Institute for Health and Clinical Excellence (NICE) and foundation hospitals. But these changes are outside the scope of this book.

Over the 50 years or so since the foundation of the RCGP, general practitioners' practice list sizes have fallen, the average number of doctors in a partnership has risen, the number of salaried doctors has increased and there has been an explosion in the number of practice staff, all fulfilling different roles. Increasingly, care is devolved into primary care. This trend will continue as we see GPs with special interests and the formation of intermediate care. Meanwhile, the number of healthcare professionals able to prescribe is steadily rising. In many cases, the traditional points of demarcation between pharmacists and GPs, or between nurses and GPs, have faded, creating overlapping roles, unlike the schisms of the seventeenth century.

From the days of the earliest healers to the modern primary care-led NHS, prescribing has been a central area in medical knowledge. This volume is aimed at those health professionals who want to build a broad foundation of prescribing principles. However, reflecting on this chapter reveals to us as prescribers how we take our place in a tradition that stretches back over the millennia.

References

1. Jackson R. *Doctors and Diseases in the Roman Empire*. 1st ed. London: British Museum Press, 1988.
2. Shapiro AK and Shapiro E. *The Powerful Placebo*. Baltimore, MD: Johns Hopkins University Press, 1997.
3. Duffin J and Campling BG. Therapy and disease concepts: The history (and future?) of antimony in cancer. *J His Med* 2002; **57**: 61–78.
4. Reeves C. *Egyptian Medicine*. 1st ed. Princes Risborough, Bucks: Shire Books, 1992.
5. Karenberg A and Leitz C. Headache in magical and medical papyri of ancient Egypt. *Cephalagia* 2001; **21**: 911–16.
6. El-Gammal SY. The role of Hippocrates in the development and progress of medical sciences. *Bull Indian Inst Hist Med Hyderabad* 1993; **23**: 125–36.
7. Manolidis LS. Otorhinolaryngology through the works of Hippocrates. *ORL J Otorhinolaryngol Relat Spec* 2002; **64**:152–6.
8. Chambers DW. A brief history of conflicting ideals in health care. *J Am Coll Dent* 2001; **68**: 48–51.
9. Kyle DG. *Spectacles of Death in Ancient Rome*. London: Routledge, 2001.
10. Sneader W. The prehistory of psychotherapeutic agents. *J Psychopharmacol* 1990; **4**: 115–19.
11. Provencal P. The Arabic pharmacology and the introduction to Europe: The background of the Arabic pharmacology – the legacy from Greece. *Dan Medicinhist Arbog* 2001; **10**: 52–70.
12. Alvarez Millan C. Graeco-Roman case histories and their influence on medieval Islamic clinical accounts. *Soc Hist Med* 1999; **12**: 19–43.
13. Al-Othman A, Al-Awad N and Parashar SK. Surgeons and the operating theater: Past, present and future. *Annals Saudi Medicine* 1998; **18**: 39–41.
14. Dunn PM. Avicenna (AD 980–1037) and Arabic perinatal medicine. *Arch Dis Child Fetal Neonatal Ed* 1997; **77**: F75–6.
15. Angeletti LR. Transmission of classical medical texts through languages of the Middle-East *Med Secoli* 1990; **2**: 293–329.
16. Laudan I. Birth of the modern diet. *Scientific American*. August 2000: 62–7.
17. Jackson WA. *The Victorian Chemist and Druggist*. 1st ed. Princes Risborough, Bucks: Shire Publications, 1996.
18. Drews J. *In Quest of Tomorrow's Medicines*. 1st ed. New York: Springer, 1999.
19. Drews J. Drug discovery: A historical perspective. *Science* 2000; **287**: 1960–4.
20. Tan Y-T, Tillett DJ and McKay IA. Molecular strategies for overcoming antibiotic resistance in bacteria. *Molecular Medicine Today* 2000; **6**: 309–14.
21. Vane JR. The fight against rheumatism: From willow bark to COX-1 sparing drugs. *J Physiol Pharmacol* 2000; **51**: 573–86.
22. Mann CC and Plummer ML. *The Aspirin Wars*. New York: Alfred A. Knopf, 1991.
23. Great Britain, Ministry of Health and Department of Health for Scotland. *A National Health Service*. London: HMSO, 1944. Cmnd 6502.

The principles of pharmacology

2

Brian Crichton

This chapter introduces some key concepts in pharmacology that all prescribers can use to place their prescribing on a more secure scientific basis. A short chapter, such as this, cannot hope to be comprehensive. It will, however, endeavour to sketch out some of the key themes underlying the principles of prescribing.

So what is pharmacology? According to Rang *et al.*[1] pharmacology is 'the study of the effects of chemical substances on the function of living systems'. In the discipline's early days, pharmacologists described drugs' biological effects, such as the fact that adrenaline contracts certain muscles. As the discipline developed, pharmacologists began to understand how chemicals exert their effects: adrenaline binds to adrenergic receptors, for example.

The next question must be 'What is a drug?' This seemingly simple question is in reality quite complex! This is due to the fact that many drugs are used in everyday living, e.g. caffeine, alcohol and nicotine. This sometimes makes it difficult to decide what a drug is and what a food is, and, as we know, many millions of pounds are spent each year on food supplements such as vitamins and minerals. Furthermore, it is known that many preparations available in health food shops contain an array of active biological molecules, which are poorly understood in terms of their actions. Despite these difficulties, a simple definition of a drug is 'a substance used in the diagnosis, treatment, or prevention of a disease or as a component of a medication'.

How do drugs work?

To understand how drugs basically work one must be reminded how naturally occurring systems work. A good example would be the hormone insulin. This peptide hormone can bind only to a specific receptor type, as both have unique shapes (see Figure 2.1). This has been likened to a lock and key, and hence 'the lock and key' hypothesis. Drugs are designed to be similar shapes to the 'keys'. They will bind to the 'lock' (receptor) but can have varying effects on it, i.e. open it (agonise) or keep it locked (antagonise).

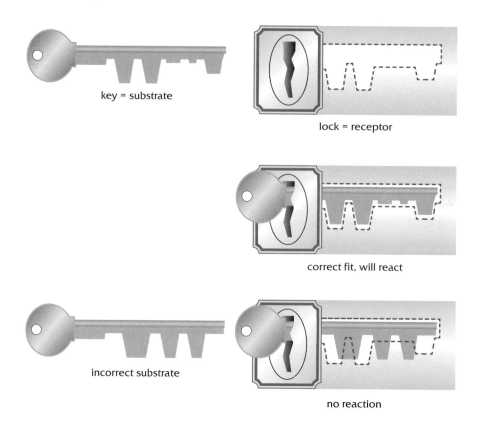

key = substrate

lock = receptor

correct fit, will react

incorrect substrate

no reaction

Figure 2.1: Lock and key hypothesis

Pharmacologists are beginning to understand the subtle biochemical and molecular intracellular pathways that translate the binding of a drug to a receptor embedded in the cell membrane to the outcome, such as muscle contraction. This increasing sophistication allows researchers to develop treatments targeted at specific molecules acting at key stages in these pathways. As we saw in Chapter 1, our understanding of non-steroidal anti-inflammatory drugs (NSAIDs) moved from a description of the effects of a herbal remedy to drugs targeted at a specific isozyme (COX-2).

Modern pharmacology can be divided into numerous disciplines (see Figure 2.2). Pharmacokinetics describes the way in which the body handles drugs (drug metabolism), for example. It can be defined as 'the study of the effects of the body on the drug, as it travels through the body'. Molecular pharmacology, as the name suggests, aims to understand a drug's action at a molecular level. As the discipline is so broad, pharmacologists often specialise in a particular system, such as the respiratory, cardiovascular or immune system.

Pharmacology impacts on many disciplines, whilst this book considers prescribing by healthcare professionals. As a result, the book focuses on clinical pharmacology. Nevertheless, depending on the discipline, other aspects could be relevant. For instance, GPs and pharmacists on formulary committees in hospitals and primary care organisation boards need to consider pharmacoeconomics, the study of the economics of prescribing (see Chapter 8). Many nurses will increasingly educate patients on how to use the products of biotechnology, such as self-injection with insulin etc. Today, one in four new drugs is a product of biotechnology.

Pharmacists are already the NHS's resident experts on pharmaceutical sciences, advising on alternative formulations in patients with swallowing difficulties following a stroke, for example. Nevertheless, in the remainder of this chapter we will focus on the main principles of clinical pharmacology, beginning with the sites of drug action.

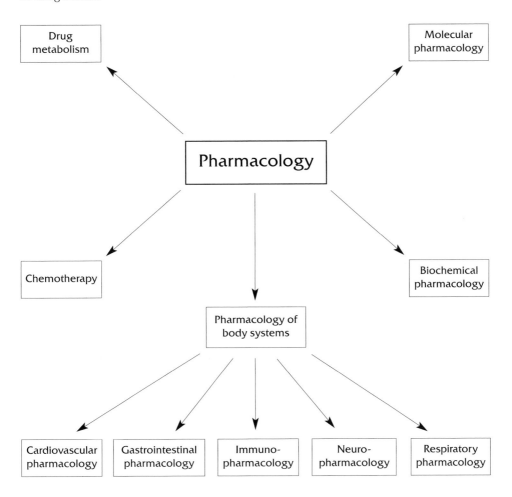

Figure 2.2: Subdivisions of pharmacology

Targeting therapeutics

As you may recall from Chapter 1, Paul Ehrlich devised the idea of a magic bullet: a drug that specifically affects abnormal tissue or an invading organism while leaving the other tissues untouched. However, a magic bullet needs a target, which either blocks (antagonises) or stimulates (agonises) a response.

Ehrlich also commented that a drug would not work unless it binds. There are exceptions to this rule – osmotic laxatives, antacids and metal chelators, for example. Nevertheless, the general principle applies to most pharmaceuticals. Indeed, current drugs target a relatively small number of molecular targets – some 483 for all the drugs marketed in the year 1996. Several different drugs can, of course, hit the same target – just think of the large number of NSAIDs, for example. However, the number of possible targets is set to increase dramatically in the wake of the Human Genome Project (HGP). As researchers work out the biological role of gene products (so-called functional genomics), numerous new enzymes, receptors and other targets are set to emerge. How many of these turn out to be suitable targets remains to be seen, but there will certainly be more than at present.

Some drugs inhibit enzymes. ACE (angiotensin-converting enzyme) inhibitors, for example, target a key enzyme in the renin-angiotensin system, which plays a central role in controlling blood pressure. Some antibodies and other protein-based drugs (the biopharmaceuticals) can bind to and inhibit cytokines (proteins that carry messages between cells). Anti-Tumour Necrosis Factor (Anti-TNF) agents have proven to be a major advance in severe rheumatoid arthritis, inflammatory bowel disease and related conditions. These bind and, therefore, deactivate this pro-inflammatory cytokine.

On balance, receptors remain the commonest drug target – as Table 2.1 shows. So to exemplify the principles of drug action, this section focuses on receptor-mediated effects.

Table 2.1: **Molecular targets of drug action – 1996 data**

Target	%
Receptors	45
Enzymes	28
Hormones and factors	11
Ion channels	5
DNA	2
Nuclear receptors	2
Unknown	7

Source: Adapted with permission from Drews J. Drug discovery: A historical perspective. *Science* 2000; **287**: 1960–4. Copyright 2000 AAAS.

Pharmacologists classify receptors into four broad 'super-families', partly based on their structure, genomic sequence, binding characteristics and so on.[1] Drug receptors can perhaps be defined as molecules with which a drug first interacts to eventually affect biological function. There is often a strict structural requirement for this interaction. Some pharmacologists prefer the term 'drug targets' and reserve the term 'receptor' to describe the macro-molecules that serve as receptors for endogenous substances. Drug targets include receptors for endogenous substances (neurotransmitters, hormones, etc.), enzymes, transport proteins, ion channels, etc.

Types of receptor

Ionotropic receptors

These are linked to ion channels, acting within a few milliseconds of the drug's binding. The binding changes the flow of ions across the cell membrane. This alters the cell's electrical state, for example propagating or blocking nerve transmission or leading to muscle contraction or relaxation. So some muscle relaxants – such as pancuronium – used during anaesthesia antagonise an ionotropic (nicotinic) receptor. Nicotinic receptors usually bind to acetylcholine, a neurotransmitter. This is, therefore, the receptor's endogenous ligand. Another ionotropic receptor – gamma-aminobutyric acid type A ($GABA_A$) – is the site of action of, for example, benzodiazepines, barbiturates, ethanol and anaesthetics. These act by binding to allosteric sites: a different region on the receptor that changes the shape of the active site (the area that actually binds the endogenous transmitter). GABA is the main inhibitory neurotransmitter in the central nervous system (CNS).

Metabotropic receptors

These are linked to G proteins (see p. 15) and can take several seconds to produce their effects. Muscarinic receptors, one example of a metabotropic receptor, also bind acetylcholine. Muscarinic agonists – such as pilocarpine – reduce intraocular pressure and, therefore, may be effective in glaucoma. Beta-adrenergic receptors are also metabotropic and are the site of action of salbutamol and other beta-adrenergic bronchodilators.

Kinase-linked receptors

These receptors are associated with an enzyme – a kinase – that phosphorylates proteins. This class of receptor can take several minutes to produce its effect. Insulin as well as many growth factors and cytokines act by binding to a kinase-linked receptor. Growth factors, as their name suggests, stimulate cells to divide. Cytokines are proteins that carry messages between cells, such as those in the immune system.

Intracellular nuclear receptors

Ionotropic, metabotropic and kinase-linked receptors all span the cell membrane. As their name suggests, however, intracellular nuclear receptors are found inside the cell, where they influence gene transcription. This means that drugs acting on intracellular nuclear receptors change the balance (i.e. the pattern of expression) of proteins produced by the genome. (Researchers refer to the proteins expressed by the genome as the proteome.) Mineralocorticoids (e.g. the hormone cortisol) and glucocorticoids (e.g. the hormone aldosterone) partly act by binding to intracellular nuclear receptors. Another group of intracellular nuclear receptors – the peroxisome proliferator-activated receptors (PPARs) – is the site of action of fibrates and thiazolidinediones (rosiglitazone and pioglitazone), used in the management of abnormal lipid profiles and Type 2 diabetes respectively.

This array of receptors allows the body to respond over a variety of time courses, from milliseconds to several hours. The various receptors will naturally influence the time course of therapeutic action. Inhaled steroids, for example, do not act quickly enough to alleviate acute asthma. Steroids take several hours to alter the balance of proteins produced by the cells in the lung from a pro-inflammatory to anti-inflammatory state. In contrast, the beta-adrenergic bronchodilators start to relax the smooth muscle surrounding the bronchioles within seconds.

Second-messenger systems

Once the agonist or antagonist binds to the target, how does this produce the effect on tissue? Antagonists bind to the receptor (or target) and block the interaction with endogenous ligand (a naturally occurring chemical that binds to the intended receptor), such as the neurotransmitter. But this raises the question: what intracellular processes does the receptor antagonist prevent?

The biochemical pathways – the so-called second-messenger systems – inside the cell that link membrane receptors with the machinery that produce the cellular effect are diverse, complex and the subject of intense research (for more information see Hancock 1997[2]). However, by way of an introduction, we will briefly examine some typical second-messenger systems.

First, for example, nerves, cardiac and skeletal muscles express voltage-gated ion channels. These open when the surrounding membrane depolarises, which allows the influx of sodium, calcium, potassium and so on. These voltage-gated ion channels are targets for a number of important drugs: for instance calcium channel blockers and local anaesthetics act by blocking calcium and sodium voltage-gated ionotropic receptors respectively. Similarly, sulphonylureas, used to treat Type 2 diabetes, seem to stimulate insulin secretion by blocking potassium channels. Moreover, mutations in ion channels seem to influence therapeutic response as well as being pathogenic in some cases of migraine, epilepsy and other diseases.

Second, metabotropic receptors are linked to 'G proteins'. G proteins, meaning guanine nucleotide binding proteins, are a family of proteins involved in second-messenger cascades. They are named thus because of their signalling mechanism, which uses the exchange of guanine diphosphate for guanine triphosphate as a general molecular 'switch' function to regulate cell processes. When an endogenous ligand or agonist binds to the metabotropic receptor, part of the protein detaches and activates the intracellular target, such as an ion channel or enzyme. In the latter case, each enzyme activated by the G protein activates many other intracellular messengers, which dramatically amplifies the signal.

Metabotropic receptors are important in many of the pathological processes contributing to diseases managed in primary care. Some G proteins, for example, activate an enzyme called phospholipase A. This enzyme modulates production of the prostaglandins contributing to inflammation. Salbutamol and sumatriptan are used to manage asthma and migraine respectively. Salbutamol and sumatriptan bind to beta-2 and $5HT_{1D/1B}$ receptors respectively. In these cases, the G proteins linked to these metabotropic receptors inhibit an enzyme called adenylate cyclase. As a final example of the importance of metabotropic receptors in clinical practice, some bacterial toxins, including those released by cholera and pertussis, are poisonous because they over-stimulate certain G proteins.

Kinase-linked receptors offer the final example of the second-messenger systems. One end of the kinase receptor binds to the ligand, such as insulin, cytokine or growth factor. When the ligand binds, the kinase phosphorylates certain amino acids that make up the receptor protein. This 'autophosphorylation' allows the receptor to interact with other enzymes inside the cell, thereby amplifying the signal.

Again, dysfunctional kinase-linked receptors contribute to a number of diseases. For example, mutated proteins, in signalling pathways controlled by kinase-linked receptors, probably contribute to several cancers by allowing the pathway to remain active even when the endogenous ligand is not bound. Many drugs targeting this important signalling pathway are in development. For example, tyrosine kinase inhibitors are marketed in some parts of the world for non-small cell lung cancer and chronic myeloid leukaemia.

Steroids and other drugs that act by binding to intracellular receptors work through a different mechanism. Cortisol (hydrocortisone) and aldosterone cross cell membranes and bind to glucocorticoid and mineralocorticoid receptors respectively. Accessory proteins associated with these receptors ensure the structure is optimal for the steroid's binding. These dissociate when the steroid binds and the complex of receptor and hormone migrates to the nucleus. Once in the nucleus, the complex binds to specific DNA sequences that change the proteins produced by the cell. This results in the clinical response. However, certain steroids – including vitamin D3, thyroid hormones and aldosterone – produce some of their effect by binding to specific membrane receptors. These are the so-called 'non-genomic' effects.[3] Molecular pharmacologists are still working out the exact clinical and therapeutic significance of these non-genomic pathways.

The dose–response relationship

Pharmacologists use a variety of mathematical models to describe the way drugs bind to their target and then produce their effect. The commonest model, known as the dose–response relationship, has a long history. In the fifteenth and sixteenth centuries, mercury was widely used to treat syphilis, although the metal caused numerous side effects ranging from hair loss to fatal kidney damage. However, there was no theoretical framework to guide prescribing until 1530, when the Swiss physician Paracelsus argued that carefully measured doses of mercury compounds taken internally could counter syphilis. Paracelsus also recognised that an excessive dose of anything could prove fatal. This formed the foundation of the dose–response relationship. As an aside, mercury used to be called quack silver and it is from this name that doctors have been termed 'quacks'.

The dose–response relationship reflects three key pharmacological principles. First, binding to receptors or other targets produces the response. Second, the concentrations of drug in the *in vivo* or *in vitro* solution surrounding the receptor determine the number of receptors bound. Third, the greater a drug's affinity for a receptor, the lower the concentration needed to occupy a given proportion of receptors.[1] The figure below shows the typical dose–response relationship for a drug binding to a receptor (Figure 2.3).

The dose–response relationship is a sigmoid. At low doses, the agonist or endogenous ligand occupies too few receptors to produce a measurable response. Above a certain threshold, the extent of binding and, therefore, the response is proportional to the concentration. The slope of the linear portion of the sigmoid relationship depends on the drug's potency. The more potent the agonist the steeper the line. At the top of the curve, the receptors are fully occupied (saturated). Therefore, once the dose–response relationship reaches a plateau, increasing the agonist concentration does not produce any further increase in response.

When prescribing, drugs tend to be used on the linear portion of the dose–response curve. So doubling, for instance, the dose of the drug will usually produce a clinically relevant increase in response. However, there comes a point where increasing the drug dosage will have no effect as the target is saturated.

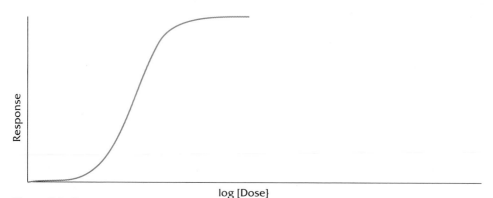

Figure 2.3: Dose–response curve

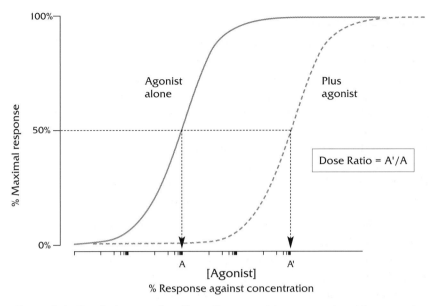

Figure 2.4: Graph showing the effect of a competitive antagonist with an agonist

Pharmacologists also use the dose–response relationship to characterise the effect of an antagonist. In the presence of a given concentration of antagonist, a higher dose of agonist or ligand is needed to evoke the same response. As a result, the dose–response curve shifts to the right (see Figure 2.4). From Figure 2.4 it can be seen that the addition of an antagonist necessitates an increase in concentration of agonist from A to A[1] in order to achieve 50 per cent of maximum response.

Of course, there are many subtleties and variations in the pattern of binding; for example, there are inverse and partial agonists, and competitive, non-competitive and insurmountable antagonists. Some biologically active drugs show 'U' shaped dose–response curves. Consideration of these types of binding is outside the remit of this volume. However, Rang *et al*. explore some of these in more detail.[1]

The therapeutic window

It is not appropriate to use the highest dose of an agonist or antagonist. Few drugs are totally specific to a particular tissue or target. So using a high dose leaves sufficient unbound drug to activate or block other receptors. In some cases, different tissues express the same receptor (although the details of the intracellular signalling system may differ). In other cases, the drug is pharmacologically 'dirty'; in other words it binds to other classes of receptor. Tricyclic antidepressants, for example, can also bind to cholinergic receptors. All these mechanisms mean that drugs can produce side effects when given at a high enough dose. However, because various classes of receptors have different affinities for the drug, the shape of dose–response varies.

A hypothetical example illustrates this principle. The linear portion of the dose–response curve for a new drug means that it is effective between 1 and 10 mg daily. Clinically significant side effects emerge between 7 and 20 mg. The dose between 1 and 7 mg is known as the therapeutic window. In other words, the dose is effective, but doesn't cause clinically significant side effects. Above 7 mg adverse effects emerge. At this point, the prescriber needs to balance the risks against the benefits.

Patients can tolerate different doses of drugs before the side effects become intolerable. Partly, this is psychological: people may be more willing to tolerate side effects if they perceive a considerable benefit from treatment. However, genetically determined differences in, for example, receptors and second-messenger systems can also contribute to the likelihood of developing side effects. As a result, patients taking some drugs – such as warfarin – require differing doses to achieve the same desired effect.

Pharmacokinetics: drugs on the move

When the patient takes the drug that has been prescribed, it is absorbed from the gut or the site of injection, distributed around the body, metabolised and excreted in bile, urine, faeces or breast milk. Pharmacokinetics offers a mathematical model of the relationship between the drug concentrations in different parts of the body during these stages of absorption, metabolism, distribution and excretion. (Pharmacodynamics, in contrast, describes the events that arise once the drug binds to its target.)

A detailed understanding of pharmacokinetics is not really needed for most prescribers. It is more important when pharmacologists try to understand a drug's characteristics during phase I studies (see Chapter 3). However, some key concepts are worth bearing in mind when perusing the prescribing literature.

For example, after a drug is administered the blood levels rise rapidly to a peak concentration (C_{max}) within a certain time (T_{max}). The peak concentration is not usually very important therapeutically. However, C_{max} can be responsible for causing some side effects.

T_{max} is more important from a clinical perspective. A drug with a short T_{max} will, in general, act more rapidly. However, it is important to remember that T_{max} is the time until the drug reaches the peak concentration in the plasma. So in the case of, for example, kinase-linked or intracellular nuclear receptors the onset of therapeutic effect may lag several minutes or hours behind T_{max}.

Drugs once absorbed are distributed amongst the body compartments, then metabolised and finally excreted. The elimination half-life ($t_{1/2}$) represents the time for the blood concentration to halve. The elimination half-life is critical in defining the dosing interval for a particular drug. A long $t_{1/2}$ – say 24 hours – may allow once-daily dosing. A shorter half-life may mean twice or thrice times daily dosing. However, the duration of action may not depend entirely on $t_{1/2}$ – the formulation is also important. As their name suggests controlled-release formulations dispense the active drug over time. This means that even drugs with a short $t_{1/2}$ can be administered once daily, as is the case with, for instance, some antihypertensives.

Finally, few drugs are administered once. Rather, repeated dosing means that the drug will accumulate until the rate of absorption matches the rate of excretion. As a rule of thumb, this is three or four times the $t_{1/2}$. So it takes between three and four days for blood levels of a once daily to reach steady state, e.g. digoxin.

Pharmacologists can describe the pattern of these changes in terms of imaginary compartments in the body. So it is possible to come across one-, two- or three-compartment models of a drug's action. However, a detailed discussion of these is again outside the scope of this book.

Metabolism and interactions

Metabolism and the related topic of drug interactions are the final pharmacological principles that we will consider in this chapter. Drugs can be metabolised in various ways. Perhaps the most important to prescribers is a group of enzymes known as the cytochrome p450 family, which are expressed in the liver and, to a lesser extent, many other tissues. Enzymes in this family form a pink compound with carbon monoxide. The colorimetric absorption of this compound peaks around 450nm – hence p450. Cyto refers to cell and chrome to colour.

Cytochrome p450 enzymes are found throughout the animal kingdom – and humans are no exception. Indeed, humans express a large number of cytochrome p450 enzymes. These have overlapping specificities for drugs and other chemicals in the environment (so-called xenobiotics). As a result, the body does not need to generate new enzymes each time it encounters a new toxin in food or the environment. The overlapping specificities allow the liver to deal with most of the environmental toxins it is likely to encounter.

The cytochromes are divided into several classes based on their genetics, proprieties and structure. In humans, cytochrome p450s are divided into three gene families, each of which contain several isozymes. So cytochrome p450 isozyme A1 of the first gene family is known as CYP1A1. Another example of an isozyme is CYP1A2 and so on and so forth.

To complicate matters further, genetic factors influence the levels of the isozymes expressed, and variations in the structure can influence both specificity and activity. For example, low levels of certain isozymes may mean that the drug is not metabolised as effectively as in the general population. As a result, the effect might be prolonged and the risk of adverse drug reactions is increased. Of course, the converse also applies. Some patients have an ultra-rapid metabolism so that they will not respond to the usual dose of some drugs. Researchers are now using genetic testing to determine the enzyme profile expressed by patients to try to predict response and the risk of side effects, especially with toxic drugs (a technique called pharmacogenomics or pharmacogenetics). A good example of this is codeine, which is metabolised to its active drug, morphine. This metabolism is dependent on CYP2D6 where some patients have very low, normal or high levels. Individuals with low levels (10 per cent of Caucasians, 1 per cent of Asians[4]) will have a poor analgesic effect from codeine whilst those with high levels (18 per cent of Saudi Arabians, 10 per cent of northern Spanish[4]) may have increased adverse events.

Effects on isozymes underlie many of the drug–drug interactions that complicate prescribing. For example, certain drugs – such as barbiturates, griseofulvin and many antiepileptics – increase production of certain isozymes. These 'inducers' increase the rate of metabolism of the other drugs metabolised by the same cytochromes. This effect can complicate the use of certain drugs such as warfarin and oral contraceptives; the induced isozyme can reduce efficacy. When the patient stops taking the inducers, plasma levels of the concurrent drug increase. As a result, the patient may experience side effects.

Moreover, the body produces a limited amount of each isozyme. So a drug that binds to one isozyme reduces the amount available to metabolise concurrent drugs. This results in increased blood levels, an enhanced effect and a greater risk of side effects.

Patients can also experience drug–drug interactions through a number of other mechanisms, as follows.

Pharmacodynamic interactions

Some drugs have similar or opposite (i.e. agonist or antagonist) effects on the same receptor. The interaction of monoamine oxidase inhibitors (a class of antidepressant) with tyramine (found in high levels in certain foods, beverages and other medications) can cause dangerous increases in blood pressure. Also, the increased likelihood of drowsiness in people who combine H_1 receptor antagonists with alcohol is another example of a pharmacodynamic interaction.

Effects on absorption

Some drugs influence the absorption of the concurrent agent. This effect is rarely clinically significant. Indeed, it can be beneficial. Local anaesthetics are often combined with adrenaline. As adrenaline contracts blood vessels, it slows absorption of the anaesthetic and prolongs the duration of action.

Changes in protein binding

Many drugs bind to proteins that circulate in blood. When more than 90 per cent of a dose of drug is bound, a concurrent agent can displace the drug and increase plasma levels. The increase is often short lived, however. The increased levels tend to stimulate greater elimination.

Altering excretion by the kidneys

Some drugs are eliminated by filtration and secretion by the kidneys. If two drugs compete for the same active transport mechanism, blood concentrations can rise. For example, some NSAIDs and methotrexate – a drug used in cancer management and severe rheumatoid arthritis – are transported by the same system. So concurrent administration can raise methotrexate levels sufficiently to cause side effects.

Many potential drug interactions arise from theoretical considerations or are implicated in case histories. Whether these interactions are clinically significant depends on the therapeutic window. If a drug is well tolerated, such as many antibiotics, even a large increase in plasma concentration is likely to be benign.

It is very difficult to predict the clinical significance of drug–drug interactions based on first principles. Indeed, chemicals in some foods and drinks – including Brussels sprouts and grapefruit juice – are metabolised by the same cytochrome (CYP) isozymes that break down some medicines. So it is important to be familiar with the possible interactions with any of the drugs you prescribe. Some adverse effects may be predictable through understood mechanisms. However, some occur where the mechanism is unknown and these reactions are called 'idiosyncratic'. The data sheet of any given drug stipulates the possible and known interactions. There is also a comprehensive list at the back of the *British National Formulary* (BNF). If there is any doubt it is advisable to check.

In this chapter, we briefly considered some of the key principles underlying clinical pharmacology. Understanding these principles places prescribing on a more rational and scientific basis. Readers needing more information about specific subjects should consult one of the excellent textbooks (e.g. Rang,[1] Hollinger[5]).

References
1. Rang HP, Dale MM, Ritter JM *et al. Pharmacology*. 5th ed. Edinburgh: Churchill Livingstone, 2003.
2. Hancock JT. *Cell Signalling*. 1st ed. Harlow: Prentice Hall, 1997.
3. Lösel R, Feuring M and Wehling M. Non-genomic aldosterone action: From the cell membrane to human physiology. *Journal of Steroid Biochemistry and Molecular Biology* 2003; **83**: 167–71.
4. Chang G and Kam P. The physiological role of cytochrome P450 isoenzymes. *Anaesthesia* 1999; **54**: 42–50.
5. Hollinger MA. *Introduction to Pharmacology*. 2nd ed. London: Taylor & Francis, 2003.

Chapter 3

Drug development – 'bench to marketplace'

Brian Crichton

Biochemical and pharmacological research is the life-blood of modern medicine. It encapsulates the very essence of human endeavour as we stride forwards in the treatment of human illness. This chapter briefly summarises the processes through which a new molecule is developed and then tested in clinical trials. It helps us to understand the basics of the regulatory requirements needed to get a drug licensed. Then, building on this knowledge, some aspects of the marketing of drugs by the pharmaceutical industry are considered.

Developing a new molecule

Pharmaceutical companies begin drug development by identifying an unmet therapeutic need. In some cases, the company may identify a disease without a currently effective treatment. In other cases, they identify conditions where the therapy is either relatively ineffective or in which the treatment often causes unacceptable side effects.[1] In general, however, the therapeutic needs tend to be those in the major markets of the developed, industrialised world rather than on an objective assessment based on medical epidemiology. For example, some 1233 new drugs were launched between 1975 and 1997. Only 13 were specifically for tropical diseases.[2] In some cases the company will develop a drug that offers a relatively small improvement over the existing agents – these are the so-called 'me-toos'.

The basic science is performed either by the pharmaceutical company itself or academics. Researchers identify a target that could potentially meet a therapeutic need: a particular receptor subtype or a specific enzyme, for example. Then they develop chemicals or proteins that bind to the target and either stimulate the biological pathways or block them. It sounds straightforward but, in reality, drug development is complex, time consuming and costly – an issue considered further later in the chapter.

Much of the costs associated with drug development arise from the considerable testing a potential new medicine undergoes before it reaches the market. For example, once researchers identify a chemical or protein (drug) that modulates a biological function, they need to quantify the drug's safety in animals and humans. As we'll see later, it's the assessment of safety and toxicity that drives the huge costs of bringing a drug to market.

So how do pharmaceutical companies identify potential new chemicals? Traditionally, chemists isolated chemicals from plants or other organisms, such as certain bacteria. Aspirin, digitalis, theophylline, quinine, Taxol (paclitaxel) and many other cancer drugs are either directly isolated from, or are chemical modifications of, plant-based chemicals. In other cases, researchers look in databases and company records for chemicals that have a similar biological action but were either ineffective or too toxic for other indications. Chemists then alter the chemical structure to, they hope, produce new agents with more activity, greater selectivity or less toxicity. The recent development of 'high-throughput screening' techniques (see below) dramatically increased demand for novel chemicals. As a result, an increasing number of pharmaceutical companies are using chemicals derived from nature once again, as a starting point for new drug development. One must remember that nature has, over millions of years of evolution, developed a remarkably diverse chemical library.

Increasingly, pharmaceutical companies also invest in powerful computer systems that allow them to model the shape of the active site of an enzyme or receptor. This allows the company to develop chemicals that, in theory at least, fit exactly into the active site producing the desired effect. However, these are only leads and any molecule developed by computer modelling still needs to be tested in animals and humans (*in vivo*). Nevertheless, computer modelling increases the likelihood that the drug will be active in the system under scrutiny.

Once chemists develop a drug or protein with the 'right' chemical characteristics, it is tested for its biological actions. Currently, biochemists and pharmacologists do not understand enough about biological systems to predict if a particular drug or protein (called a biopharmaceutical) will have the desired effect *in vivo*. So, unfortunately, there is no reasonable substitute for testing the agent in anything other than real tissue.

So, for example, researchers might use a piece of tissue with a well-understood biochemistry and physiology, such as a section of a guinea pig's intestine isolated in an organ bath, to test the drug. Pharmacologists know which drugs make the muscles in the intestine contract and by adding various antagonists they can selectively block or activate a variety of receptors. This allows them to confirm that, for example, the drug binds to a particular receptor subtype. The effect of the various established agonists and antagonists, as well as the extent of the contraction produced or inhibited, offers researchers an insight into the agent's affinity and selectivity. In a more sophisticated approach, researchers may use radioactively tagged (radiolabelled) chemicals to quantify the drug's binding characteristics. After testing on several tissues, the pharmacologist moves to live animal experiments. In some cases, detailed tissue work may be inappropriate and researchers need to move directly to animals.

Another *in vitro* model uses a layer of cells grown in flat-bottomed bottles – a technique known as cell culture. Drugs that kill the cells may be toxic, for example. (Although this might be exactly the response sought by researchers looking for new cancer drugs.) Researchers can add biological chemicals, such as cytokines (proteins that carry messages between cells), and examine the effect of a new anti-inflammatory or cancer treatment that specifically targets this mediator, for example. Again, however, any hypotheses generated in cell culture need confirmation in animal and human experiments. Although cell culture offers some important insights, a layer of cells is not analogous to a complex biological system, such as an organ, or even a human!

Until recently, determining whether a new chemical binds to a specific receptor or enzyme was time consuming. Researchers could only, at best, test a few samples each day. However, a new approach – called high-throughput screening – dramatically increases the number of new assays researchers can perform, from around 10,000 to 100,000 annually. New generations of high-throughput screens could increase the number of samples to 100,000 per day! Clearly, high-throughput screening dramatically increases the chances of a 'hit'. This advance is set to become especially important with the sequencing of the human genome, which is set to yield a vast number of receptors, enzymes and other therapeutic targets.

None of these techniques accurately mimics the subtleties of complex intact organs. As a result, animal research is a prerequisite for clinical trials and offers important insights into whether a drug may be safe and effective in humans. In some cases – such as certain mechanisms controlling blood pressure – the animal's physiology is close enough to humans to assess efficacy and toxicity. In other cases, researchers use a so-called 'model' of a disease that doesn't have an equivalent in animals. For instance, researchers can now breed animals that express, for example, proteins characteristic of some brain disorders or certain genes. This allows researchers to look at the new drug's action on the biochemical abnormality. Nevertheless, some conditions are difficult to model in animals, especially those such as schizophrenia, pain and depression that include cognitive and emotional elements. The best researchers can hope for is to use a surrogate marker for the effect.

Nevertheless, as everyone reading this book is well aware, using animals in research is fraught with ethical issues. Although everyone using pharmaceuticals should be aware of the comments, the debate is too complex to summarise here. However, Bernard Rollin's[3] and Peter Singer's[4] books offer thought-provoking introductions to the issues.

Some points are worth highlighting, however. First, animal research in the UK is tightly regulated under a raft of legislation. Researchers and the facilities are licensed, for example. Experiments must use the minimum number of animals and researchers must take reasonable and appropriate steps to limit pain and suffering. Moreover, animal experiments are required for a drug's licensing. This position argues that regulated animal experimentation is needed to maximise the reduction in human suffering. However, some animal rights activists hold an absolute view that it is wrong to use one being to benefit another. In the heat of the argument, both sides tend to forget that the choice between these positions is a value judgement rather than an absolute truth. Each person needs to decide for him or herself where their position lies.

Clinical studies

Once a drug has been shown to be potentially well tolerated and effective in animals, human testing can begin. The idea of comparative trials in humans dates from around the middle of the eighteenth century. Bishop and philosopher George Berkeley advocated using tar water for several ailments. Physicians dismissed the idea. So Berkeley suggested comparing tar water to a standard treatment, keeping other factors constant. However, no one seems to have performed this experiment.[5] Nevertheless, Berkeley helped establish the idea of comparative clinical trials.

The first recognisable comparative clinical study began in 1747. Scurvy (which we now know is caused by a deficiency in vitamin C) was the scourge of the Royal Navy. So James Lind allocated twelve men with scurvy to take one of the following:

- a quart of cider a day
- 25 drops of elixir vitriol three times a day
- two spoonfuls of vinegar three times a day
- half a pint of sea water a day
- a concoction of nutmeg, mustard and garlic three times a day
- or two oranges and a lemon a day.

Citrus fruits emerged as the most effective treatment. However, Lind didn't accept his findings, suggesting fresh air and a change in diet as the cure for scurvy. Shapiro and Shapiro suggest that the 'weight of tradition' might have been too much for Lind to bear.[5] Even today some effective treatments can have a difficult time entering healthcare professionals' practice partly because of this weight of tradition.

Phases of drug evaluation

Today, clinical studies performed before a drug is marketed take place in three phases. It's worth noting that only 71 per cent of the drugs in phase I enter phase II. Astoundingly, just 31.4 per cent reach phase III.[6] The drugs fail for a variety of reasons, including toxicity and lack of efficacy. This comprehensive testing regimen emerged in response to the thalidomide tragedy and the resulting emphasis on drug regulation (see p. 29). Before then, drugs could be launched with very little testing. For example, an antibiotic was introduced in 1959 following just two weeks of toxicity tests. Librium was tested on 1163 patients. However, in epilepsy just three patients received the drug in the initial studies.[7] The introduction of the three phases of pre-launch clinical trials has contributed to patient safety and better health outcomes. Nevertheless, the system is not infallible and a small number of drugs with excessive toxicity still reach the marketplace, only to be withdrawn later. This occurs mainly because of idiosyncratic reactions where the mechanism is unpredictable and may only occur once in many thousands of patients.

The phase I study

During phase I studies, a few subjects – usually young, healthy male volunteers – take the drug under tightly controlled conditions. (Women of reproductive potential tend to be excluded.) Often the volunteers remain in dedicated phase I units so that they can be continually monitored and to prevent external factors from affecting the results. The volunteers take increasing doses of the drug until side effects emerge. This is the maximum tolerated dose. Researchers measure blood pressure, heart rate, liver function and other critical physiological parameters. Phase I studies do not aim to quantify efficacy; rather they aim to characterise safety, pharmacokinetics and pharmacodynamics. In some cases – for example in the study of many cancer treatments – phase I studies enrol patients directly. It would certainly be ethically unacceptable (see below) to expose healthy people to drugs likely to be toxic.

The phase II study

During phase II studies, several hundred patients with the disease the drug is supposed to treat take the medication for a few weeks or months. The dose, however, tends to be less than the maximum tolerated dose characterised during phase I. Phase II studies allow the pharmaceutical company to better characterise safety, pharmacokinetics and pharmacodynamics in a broader, but still highly selected, population. Certain diseases, as well as factors such as sex, race or age, can alter a drug's pharmacokinetics and pharmacodynamics, for example. Phase II studies also offer the first indication of whether the drug is effective enough against the target disease to warrant further development.

The phase III study

Phase III studies are the acid test for a new drug. Phase III studies aim to quantify how effective and well tolerated the new drug will be in clinical practice. As such, phase III studies form the basis of the application to the licensing authorities needed to market the drug. In order to gain an accurate impression of the drug's efficacy and tolerability, hundreds, and in some cases many thousands, of patients – often at several centres in a number of countries – need to take the agent for a protracted period, which can last for years. The dose used is that identified during phase II.

Phase III studies ensure that broader ranges of patients are exposed to the drug, although this might not fully reflect the population in real-life practice. The test drug is often compared to a better-established treatment rather than the placebo, which tends to be used in the earlier phases. It would be ethically unacceptable to knowingly give patients a placebo for a long period of time, if an adequate treatment exists. However, even with the huge size of phase III drugs, rare side effects may not emerge until a large, unselected population uses the drug. As a result, some drugs are withdrawn after launch because of side effects.

The design of modern controlled clinical studies owes much to the work of Austin Bradford Hill, a pioneer in the use of statistics in research. Before modern antibiotics, tuberculosis (TB) was a major killer and there were few effective treatments. So when streptomycin was introduced as a treatment for TB, Hill and colleagues designed a clinical study to compare the new drug with bed rest – which was then the gold standard. Streptomycin proved its effectiveness and the study showed the benefits of a carefully designed trial employing careful clinical observation, objective evaluations and statistics.[5] The principles established in this study remain the foundation of clinical studies today.

Since Hill's pioneering work, the randomised controlled study emerged as the study design of choice, although Ronald Fisher first applied the statistical concept of randomisation, developed in 1885, to experimentation in 1926. Randomisation became common practice after he published *The Design of Experiments* in 1935. During randomised controlled studies a group of patients have an equal chance of receiving the test drug and either the placebo or comparative agent.

Whenever possible, the study is 'blinded'. In other words, patients, investigators or both do not know which treatment is which. The term 'blind' first was used in 1917. Several individuals seem to have independently developed the double-blind concept. However, blinded studies are not always practical. In open studies, the patient and clinician know which drug they are using. In some cases, the patient may switch between drugs – known as a crossover design.

Clearly, patients and physicians involved in clinical trials have rights and responsibilities. Rather than leave these to individual conscience, clinical trials are governed by a code of ethics known as the Declaration of Helsinki, formulated in 1964 and amended on several occasions.[8] The Declaration establishes a framework ensuring that, for instance, the patients' interests take precedence over those of science and society. According to the Declaration 'biomedical research involving human subjects cannot legitimately be carried out unless the importance of the objective is in proportion to the inherent risk to the subject'.

Locally, each hospital has an ethics committee that ensures any study performed under its auspices conforms to the principles established in the Declaration. So, to take one example, the ethics committee ensures that patients give 'informed consent'. The committee reviews the information provided to patients and the form that patients sign to confirm that they understand the study's nature, benefits and risks, and their own rights and responsibilities.

Clinical studies need to be performed to a high standard to ensure scientific validity and patient safety. This also ensures that the sponsoring company can use the results in their regulatory submissions. In most cases, this means that the researchers need to adhere to good clinical practice (GCP), an internationally agreed set of rules and regulations that determines standards for design, conduct, performance, monitoring, analyses and so on. To take one example, researchers follow standard operating procedures (SOPs) and work according to a detailed protocol. The sponsoring company regularly audits the researchers to ensure that they are following the protocol and that the data collected is at an acceptable standard.

The phase IV study

The final clinical trial phase takes place once the drug is licensed and reaches the marketplace. During phase IV studies, large numbers of patients – often enrolled from general practices or district general hospitals – take the medication to gain an insight into its effectiveness and safety in everyday practice. Another post-marketing study – known as safety assessment of marketed medicines (SAMM) – enrols many thousands of patients to identify rare, unexpected side effects.

Regulatory requirements

In the UK, the legal requirement for drugs to obtain marketing approval before launch followed the thalidomide tragedy. Thalidomide was marketed in the late 1950s as a sedative and a treatment for morning sickness. However, by the early 1960s it became clear that taking thalidomide during pregnancy caused severe birth defects. Eventually over 10,000 babies were affected. This disaster prompted governments worldwide to implement stringent regulations controlling the assessment of new drugs, in particular for safety. Recently, however, thalidomide emerged as a potentially effective treatment for several serious conditions, including AIDS wasting syndrome. Obviously, it is only used under close surveillance by specialists, whilst women of child-bearing potential use effective contraception.[9]

Over the years, a variety of marketing approval schemes emerged in the countries that comprise the European Union. All these scrutinise the huge amount of data generated during the animal, clinical and other experiments to ensure that the drug is both safe and effective. Moreover, the regulatory authorities ensure that manufacturing plants and processes reach certain standards. So, for example, the authorities ensure that a company has adequate strategies to recall products if a safety issue emerges.

As part of the move to increasing transparency between countries, procedures were harmonised under the European Medicines Agency (EMEA). The London-based agency opened in 1995. In some cases, companies apply directly to the EMEA for a new drug licence. In other cases, a company applies to a country's regulatory authority. Other members of the European Union should accept this decision and the EMEA mediates any disputes.

Marketing

The research and development (R&D) of a new drug is costly. For example, DiMasi and colleagues[6] estimated the pre-tax R&D costs for new drugs by surveying several pharmaceutical companies. As mentioned above, only around a fifth of drugs that begin clinical development eventually reach the market. Estimates, therefore, need to allow for the costs of developing medicines that were abandoned. Bringing a new drug to market takes an average of 72.1 months.[10] So economists include a discount rate to allow for the time scales. They also include post-approval R&D. The total cost of bringing a drug to market was found to be nearly US$900 million. This is roughly the same as the sum needed to buy a squadron of 40 F16 fighters.[11] Furthermore, pharmaceutical companies increasingly develop drugs for chronic and degenerative diseases. These are much harder to investigate than acute conditions or relatively straightforward diseases such as hypertension. As a result, R&D costs are growing at, on average, 7.4 per cent annually above general inflation.[6]

Against this background, pharmaceutical companies use several strategies to market drugs to healthcare professionals. The so-called 'below the line' promotion includes direct mail, exhibitions, point-of-sale material and free samples to health professionals. 'Above the line' advertising includes press, television, radio and posters, though direct selling to the public is prohibited in the UK. Most pharmaceutical companies sponsor medical education. Indeed, medical education in the UK would be considerably reduced if it were not for company sponsorship (see Chapter 11 for a critique!). Traditionally, medical education targets doctors. However, education and pharmaceutical marketing is increasingly engaging the growing number of stakeholders in health care – managers, patients, nurses and other professions, as well as doctors. Engaging stakeholders can be done in various ways, but an example would be the funding of disease awareness in an area that a pharmaceutical company had a particular interest.

Nevertheless, the traditional approach of persuading doctors to prescribe by combining sales representatives' visits and advertising remains the cornerstone of marketing strategies. Advertising raises prescribers' awareness of a product and aims to engender confidence in the brand. Sales representatives can then build on this confidence and awareness during their meetings with the individual prescribers. It is during these meetings that the healthcare professionals review the data supporting the claims made about the brand and need to be equipped with the ability to critically appraise (see Chapter 11).

In hospitals, representatives often discuss a single drug. However, in primary care representatives may promote several drugs in order of importance to the company. If the doctor isn't interested in the first drug, the representative moves on to the second, then the third and so on. Representatives call on a number of strategies to influence doctors. For example, the representatives may offer printed material, patient information leaflets or invitations to meetings or congresses. In the past, some promotional activities attracted considerable criticism. Today, the hospitality is secondary to the medical content[12] and strictly regulated (see below).

Another common strategy may appeal to people in authority, such as the specialists involved in the phase III studies. These 'opinion leaders' balance their independent credibility with being seen as influenced by pharmaceutical companies. So most now disclose any financial arrangements in journals and presentations. In other cases, sales representatives refer to the fact that the doctor's colleagues use the drug. Finally, if the relationship is appropriate, the representative may make a direct request to use the product or enter into a debate about the medicine's merits.[13]

The pharmaceutical representative

Despite the large number of encounters that prescribers may have had with drug representatives, it is worth asking the question, 'How well do we actually understand these professionals?' In this section we will consider the training of drug representatives and briefly look at the Association of the British Pharmaceutical Industry (ABPI).

Pharmaceutical representatives have examinations that they have to sit within the first two years of employment. The syllabus of these exams is surprisingly broad and basically consists of three parts as detailed below.

- Section 1 has four chapters that cover the topics of the NHS, the pharmaceutical industry, the ABPI and the ABPI Code of Practice (see below).

- Section 2 broadly covers the areas of the human body, pathology, the immune system and pharmacology.

- Section 3 covers the main systems, namely the circulatory, respiratory, nervous, digestive, musculoskeletal, endocrine, urinary and reproductive systems. The skin and special senses are also covered. For those specialising in female health a special supplementary paper is required.

The ABPI examination plus the individual pharmaceutical company product training (which may be many weeks long) makes representatives more highly trained than we might initially think!

Strict rules and regulations are in place for those pharmaceutical companies that are members of the ABPI, which runs as an independent organisation. A small minority are non-members, but invariably all adhere to its Code of Practice. The most common reason for not being a member is a function of the size of the pharmaceutical company. Small companies often can ill afford to release members to sit on the various steering committees that exist within the ABPI or the annual levy incumbent on its members.

The inception of the ABPI was in 1958 and the organisation has undergone many revisions since. These revisions are not carried out in isolation and occur in consultation with the British Medical Association (BMA), the Royal Pharmaceutical Society of Great Britain (RPSGB), and the Medicines and Healthcare products Regulatory Agency (MHRA) of the Department of Health. The whole ethos of the ABPI Code of Practice is to ensure that the promotion of medicines is carried out in a responsible, ethical and professional manner.[13] The ABPI has teeth if it finds a company in breach of its Code of Practice! It can apply any of a number of sanctions.

Marketing evolution

Pharmaceutical marketing is becoming increasingly sophisticated. There is a growing use of internet resources, such as dedicated password-protected sites for healthcare professionals. In some cases – such as asthma, diabetes or for the growing number of injectable biopharmaceuticals – pharmaceutical companies 'sponsor' nurses to perform specific service tasks such as running clinics or teaching patients and carers how to administer the medicine. The idea behind this is not to promote a specific drug, but supply an added service to medicine. In the case of a clinic, active screening and intervention allows a trained nurse to case-find and optimise treatment. The company accepts that some of its rivals may also benefit. The aim is to expand the market generally. In other cases – such as teaching patients how to self-inject – the sponsored nurse takes some of the workload off the shoulders of the members of the primary care teams.

Finally, it is worth mentioning that some companies are beginning to work with primary care organisations and other purchasers and providers to implement a particular strategy. In one case, a health authority collaborated with the industry to encourage prescribers to switch to a cheaper proton pump inhibitor. This released money that was invested to better manage other projects, such as heart disease.[14] Healthcare professionals can expect a growth in such innovative marketing strategies over the next few years. If carefully implemented and critically assessed, such strategies can offer a win for companies, a win for the NHS and a win for patients.

The cost of modern medicines and the activities of pharmaceutical companies attract considerable criticism from some quarters. This chapter shows that pharmaceutical R&D requires a huge amount of investment, in both time and money. Companies need to make a reasonable return on this investment. However, by taking promotion with 'a pinch of salt', by rigorously reviewing the evidence base and by applying a critical eye, the material can be a valuable resource. It is a simple fact of life that without healthcare professionals' active support, the pharmaceutical industry would no longer be able to develop the new drugs that the patients need both today and in the future.

References

1. Greener M. *A Healthy Business*. London: Informa Publishing, 2001.
2. Reich MR. The global drug gap. *Science* 2000; **287**: 1979–81.
3. Rollin BE. *The Frankenstein Syndrome*. Cambridge, UK: Cambridge University Press, 1995.
4. Singer PA. *Practical Ethics*. 2nd ed. Cambridge, UK: Cambridge University Press, 1993.
5. Shapiro AK and Shapiro E. *The Powerful Placebo*. Baltimore, MD: Johns Hopkins University Press, 1997.
6. DiMasi JA, Hansen RW and Grabowski HG. The price of innovation: New estimates of drug development costs. *Journal of Health Economics* 2003; **22**: 151–85.
7. Marks L. Human guinea pigs? The history of the early oral contraceptive clinical trials. *History and Technology* 1999; **15**: 263–8.
8. World Medical Organization. Declaration of Helsinki. *British Medical Journal* 1996; **313(7070)**: 1448–9.
9. Timmermans S and Leiter V. The redemption of thalidomide: Standardizing the risk of birth defects. *Soc Stud Sci* 2000; **30**: 41–71.
10. Keyhani S, Diener-West M and Powe N. Are development times for pharmaceuticals increasing or decreasing? *Health Affairs* 2006; **25**: 461–8.
11. Frank RG. New estimates of drug development costs. *Journal of Health Economics* 2003; **22**: 325–30.
12. Roughead EE, Harvey KJ and Gilbert AL. Commercial detailing techniques used by pharmaceutical representatives to influence prescribing. *Aust N Z J Med* 1998; **28**: 306–10.
13. *ABPI Code of Practice for the Pharmaceutical Industry*. London: ABPI, 2003.
14. Freemantle N, Johnson R, Dennis J, *et al*. Sleeping with the enemy? A randomized controlled trial of a collaborative health authority/industry intervention to influence prescribing practice. *Br J Clin Pharmacol* 2000; **49**: 174–9.

Prescribing professionals in primary care

Brian Crichton

Traditionally, GPs have always been the main primary care professionals able to prescribe medicines. Dentists were able to prescribe but from a much smaller formulary. However, until recently, no other healthcare professionals could prescribe for their patients. Nevertheless, nurses were taking on increasing responsibility for the care of their patients in diseases such as asthma and diabetes. They made *de facto* prescribing decisions within protocols and guidelines agreed by the practice, but had to find a GP to sign the script.

Clearly, this was a waste of time for both the nurse and GP as well as undermining the former's professional autonomy. Moreover, there was no compelling pharmacological reason why nurses and other healthcare professionals, appropriately trained and working to agreed guidelines and protocols, could not prescribe many medicines. Concomitantly, the rules surrounding prescribing have been progressively relaxed over recent years.

As a result, a growing number of professionals in primary care are able to prescribe a wide range of drugs, albeit under carefully controlled circumstances. The recent introduction of supplementary prescribing has the potential of dramatically increasing the number of primary care professionals able to prescribe. The professions first chosen for this have been the pharmacists and nurses, as they are numerically the largest non-medical groups and are deemed to be able to offer the greatest impact. In this chapter, we review the various groups able to prescribe. Such an expansion benefits GPs, the other professions, the NHS budget – and, most importantly, patients.

Shared care

The growing number of healthcare professionals able to prescribe obviously increases the onus on the different professionals to work together effectively and efficiently. This is especially the case when the disease is complex, complicated by concurrent conditions or involves the use of treatments with potentially problematical side effects. Of course, informal networks of healthcare professionals have long been in place. GPs and their secondary care colleagues need to communicate and work together. Nevertheless, these arrangements tended to arise *ad hoc* or be mediated on an informal basis through letters and phone calls. Inevitably, the quality of the interaction between different healthcare professionals varied markedly and, in some cases, there was a tendency to be protective over professional roles. 'Shared care' aims to put these relationships on a more formal basis as well as better demarking and developing professional roles.

More recently, a political imperative has helped to drive the tendency towards shared care. Increasingly, we are seeing healthcare reforms shift the balance of power in the NHS towards primary care. So shared care means more than working vertically across the primary and secondary care interface. Shared care means working horizontally with other members of the primary or secondary care team.

For example, a 'Managed Clinical Network' for vascular services in Lanarkshire is vertically integrated from the Health Board to the Acute Hospital Trust to the Primary Care Trust. Informal networking already existed in Lanarkshire. However, this foundation was built on by the Managed Clinical Network[1] – which should be the case in all services developing the shared-care ethos. Indeed, shared care has proven its value in numerous conditions including pulmonary arterial hypertension,[2] erectile dysfunction,[3] prostate disease[4] as well as numerous other diseases.

Apart from optimising clinical outcomes and developing and augmenting professional roles, shared care can improve cost-effectiveness, releasing funds for other services. For instance, over one year, a shared-care prostate assessment clinic run by a trained urology nurse assessed 1080 patients with suspected bladder outflow obstruction following GP referral using a standard pro forma. Around a third of patients were referred directly back to primary care. The system saved around £24,000 a year.[4]

Nevertheless, to work effectively and efficiently, a shared-care service needs to overcome several obstacles including professionals' protectiveness about their roles. The shared-care team need to be empowered, with shared philosophies and goals.[5] The issue of clinical responsibility also needs to be clearly defined and agreed.

Against this background, developing local protocols and Patient Group Directions (see below) can help clarify and codify these issues enhancing shared care. For example, a protocol for treating acute constipation in the community helped overcome the ambiguity concerning limits of the nurse's role in treating this condition. The protocol 'empowers appropriately trained community nurses' to manage adults suffering from acute constipation.[6] It is key, however, to develop such protocols locally. Those protocols with buy-in from the local stakeholders are far more likely to be implemented and accepted than a top-down approach. Local purchasers and providers can, however, use examples of best practice from other trusts and adapt these to local circumstances, supported by regular audit.

Patient Group Directions

Patient Group Directions, as their name suggests, offer specific written instructions for supplying or administering medicines to groups of patients rather than individuals. So, for example, a Patient Group Direction could cover the administration of thrombolytics by paramedics to patients with suspected heart attack. As this example suggests, Patient Group Directions should confer 'a clear, quantifiable advantage to the patient' without compromising safety. The breadth and number of these directions are gradually increasing and thus some consideration is needed at this point.

Patient Group Directions do not replace individualised care. They are used in specific circumstances, such as when the benefits of rapid intervention are likely to outweigh any risks. As such, senior doctors, pharmacists and representatives of the professions likely to contribute to care develop each Patient Group Direction. The Direction is also authorised by the employer – for example the primary care organisation. As a further safeguard, drug and therapies committees and appropriate local professional advisory committees must also approve the directives. Importantly stakeholders must agree lines of accountability, which should be clearly documented.

The Patient Group Directions allow qualified health professionals to administer a medicinal product in certain specific circumstances. Currently, the 'qualified health professionals' that can follow a Patient Group Direction include nurses, midwives, health visitors, optometrists, pharmacists, orthoptists, physiotherapists, chiropodists/podiatrists, radiographers and ambulance paramedics. Local managers maintain a register of approved staff, which has written evidence showing that they are authorised to provide care under the specific Patient Group Directions.

NHS Trusts, health boards, GP or dental practices and NHS-funded family planning clinics can develop Patient Group Directions, although controlled drugs are excluded. The regulations suggest exercising special caution before covering parenteral and antimicrobial medicines with Patient Group Directions. Furthermore, Patient Group Directions cover the following only under 'exceptional' circumstances:

- a new drug under intensive monitoring and subject to special adverse reaction reporting
- unlicensed medicines
- medicines used outside the terms of the Summary of Product Characteristics
- medicines used in the care of children.

In such cases, the Patient Group Directions need to show that patient safety is not compromised and that the procedures offer additional benefits for patients.

Against this background, each Patient Group Direction needs to offer 'a clear and unambiguous definition of the clinical condition/situation'. So the Direction should set out the criteria for confirming that, first, the patient suffers from the condition and, second, that a patient is eligible for inclusion. The Direction should also set out exclusion criteria, such as patients with complex medical needs or who are inappropriate ages. Prescribing to children can be problematical, while age-related changes in renal or hepatic handling can complicate management in the elderly. Finally, the Patient Group Direction should specify what action to take if patients do not want to receive, do not adhere to, or are excluded from care.

Each Patient Group Direction also describes several key features about the medicine, such as the legal status and dose(s), and the criteria for deciding administration method and route, frequency of administration and the maximum daily dose. The Direction should highlight advice for patients and any warnings, as well as how to identify and manage possible adverse events. Local pharmacovigilance arrangements need to be in place and all medicines have to be supplied pre-packed.

Each trust has to ensure that there are adequate records for patients treated under the Direction. There needs to be a clear audit trail and data set, including, at the very least, the health professional's name, patient community health index number, and the medicine. Ideally, patients should give written consent. If this is impossible, the healthcare professionals need to document verbal consent.

Finally, the Patient Group Direction should be reviewed at least once every two years. However, the Direction should also state criteria for interim review, as, for example, evidence changes or experience accumulates.

Training prescribing professionals
General practitioners

General practitioners are the leading prescribers of pharmaceuticals in the UK. In 2002, the Department of Health estimated that community pharmacists dispensed some 650 million prescriptions in England alone – that's almost 11 prescriptions for every man, woman and child in the UK.[7] Moreover, GPs can prescribe almost every drug in the *British National Formulary*, with a few exceptions (such as drugs that require specialist knowledge and those on the Black List).

GPs undergo extensive training to allow them to balance the risks and benefits associated with each medicine for each patient. At first sight, the large number of drugs in some areas may seem pharmaceutical overkill. There is a diverse range of non-steroidal anti-inflammatory drugs (NSAIDs) for example. However, some patients benefit from one NSAID but not another. (This diverse effect could be explained by genetically determined differences in the enzymes responsible for NSAID actions.[8]) GPs need to appreciate the diverse range of agents available to them and be *au fait* with their different pharmacological, pharmacokinetic and pharmacodynamic properties. (For an explanation of these terms see Chapter 2.)

This degree of pharmaceutical sophistication – along with the other skills needed to be an effective GP – takes considerable training. So following five years (on average) as undergraduates, medical students receive a medical degree. All doctors allowed to practise medicine are registered with the General Medical Council (GMC) after doing a pre-registration year as a junior hospital doctor subsequent to qualifying. Doctors who wish to become GPs undertake at least three years' further training, both in hospital and primary care. At the end of this time, they receive a certificate of training that allows them to work as a GP. In other words, a GP's basic training takes, on average, at least nine years.

Many GPs sit further examinations, such as those held under the auspices of the Royal College of General Practitioners (RCGP). Membership of the RCGP, for example, indicates that the GP has been assessed and considered to have expertise across the whole spectrum of general practice. Fellows of the RCGP have been members of the College for at least five years. These GPs are awarded the fellowship because they show particularly high standards of practice. The fellowship may also be awarded for services to the College and the medical profession. The MRCGP syllabus improves a doctor's ability to prescribe in many ways. It allows an individual to reflect on the very essence of the consultation and gain an understanding of consultation theory and practice. The syllabus also includes a section on critical appraisal, which enables one more confidently to identify reliable new data and research work, be discriminating in one's reading, be more consistent in using good-quality evidence in decision making and be better able to develop evidence-based services. All these facets may challenge an individual's present and future prescribing behaviour. Other postgraduate courses can also have an impact on a doctor's prescribing. Indeed, there are specifically designed courses on the area of prescribing, which can be at award, certificate, diploma or higher levels (see Chapter 11), depending on the clinician's requirements.

GPs can study for additional diplomas according to their particular interests, such as obstetrics and gynaecology, child health, family planning, geriatric medicine, occupational medicine and public health. These qualifications increase the knowledge base in their respective areas, but have no particular prescribing focus.

Nurses

The emphasis in nurse training is somewhat different from that of GPs. Even nurses who have a special interest and expertise in, for example, cancer, Parkinson's disease or asthma tend to focus on holistic patient care, rather than the clinical aspects of specific illnesses or conditions. Of course, the two are intimately linked and clinical management is an increasingly important element in nurses' skill mix. Nevertheless, nurses tend to spend more time than GPs working with patients and their families, providing care and offering health promotion, education and counselling. Midwives are specialist nurses who support the mother, baby and family through pregnancy, birth itself and postnatally.

Nurses and midwives study for three or four years, on courses run by universities that lead to either a diploma or degree. In addition to the academic training, nurses gain further skills and knowledge during placements in both primary and secondary care, the course being half-theory and half-practical. During the first year, the student nurses participate in a Common Foundation Programme, which introduces them to the basic principles of nursing. They then specialise in adult or children's nursing, mental health or learning disability nursing. Once qualified, nurses can undergo further training to become, for instance, nurse prescribers (see below). Increasingly, however, prescribing is becoming a core component of undergraduate nursing courses.

The practice nurse

To become a practice nurse, the individual should hold an appropriate qualification that is registered or recorded on the effective part of the Professional Register maintained by what was previously known as the United Kingdom Central Council for Nurses, Midwives and Health Visitors (UKCC), but now called the Nursing and Midwifery Council (NMC). The nurse will normally have a Registered General Nurse qualification. Where the practice nurse holds the qualification of an Enrolled Nurse (General), then he or she may only undertake a more limited range of duties, having due regard to the skills of enrolled nurses contained within the nurse training rules of the NMC.

The focus of the practice nurse's role is in patient education, encompassing health promotion, screening, disease prevention and chronic disease management. Further specialist training is needed to provide the nurse with the knowledge and skills necessary to fulfil the broad range of duties that are required in primary care. In particular, specialist training in diabetes and asthma is available on courses offered at diploma level and above. These courses fully equip the practice nurse with the expertise to support the GP in the management of these conditions, as most chronic disease management occurs in primary care. It is clear, however, that the role of the practice nurse is broadening as it keeps pace with the changes that are occurring in primary care. An example of this has been seen in the genesis of two new positions, each being at the opposite ends of the qualification spectrum. At the one end there is the healthcare assistant. This post requires no formal nursing qualification, though there are modular courses that can be assessed giving the individual an NVQ level 3. They can help practices with some important tasks such as phlebotomy, data collection and specific healthcare counselling (smoking cessation, weight reduction, etc.). At the other end of the spectrum is the nursing practitioner. Qualified to a minimum of degree level in specialist or advanced nursing practice, the nurse practitioner offers an expanded nursing role to the primary healthcare team. In the rapidly changing climate of health care today, nurse practitioners are expanding the boundaries of nursing and developing nursing practice. By working collaboratively with GPs in primary care, they offer patients increased access to a medical professional. Nurse practitioners are seeing patients with undifferentiated health problems, often discharging patients from care without referral to another healthcare professional. They consult with patients who have undiagnosed health problems and assess, diagnose, offer education, treatment or referrals and accept responsibility for autonomous decision making. In addition, they often initiate and manage a nursing caseload of identified patients, primarily with chronic diseases and manage their care in nurse-led clinics.

The roles of the healthcare assistant and nursing practitioner are particularly important when we consider the challenges of the data collection and chronic disease management required for the new, 2004 GP contract.

Nurse prescribing

In 1989, the Advisory Group on Nurse Prescribing suggested that nurse prescribing could improve patient care and make better use of patients', nurses' and GPs' time. The Advisory Group stated that nurse prescribing would also clarify professional responsibilities and improve communications between team members. Following successful pilots, by September 2001 over 22,000 district nurses and health visitors – including around 1000 practice nurses – had been trained to prescribe from the *Nurse Prescribers' Formulary*.[9] They carry the title of Community Practitioner Nurse Prescribers. As mentioned above, this change formalised the current relationship, where appropriately trained nurses effectively make prescribing decisions and are thus independent prescribers. The Review of Prescribing, Supply and Administration of Medicines described independent prescribers as professionals who are responsible for the initial assessment of the patient and for devising the broad treatment plan, with the authority to prescribe the medicines required as part of that plan.

In May 2001, the DoH extended the scheme to cover minor ailments and injuries, health promotion and palliative care.[9] However, further changes were put in place to enable nurses without district nursing or health visiting qualifications to prescribe from the *Nurse Prescribers' Extended Formulary*, after appropriate training. The prescribing programme includes 25 taught days in a university, plus 12 days of 'learning in practice' supervised by a medical practitioner. The end point of this course is where nurses undergo an assessment of theory and practice. Perhaps the most fundamental change of all (from 1 May 2006) has been the authorisation of Nurse Independent Prescribers to prescribe any licensed drug for any medical condition within their level of experience and competence. This includes a limited number of controlled drugs detailed in Annexe A at the end of this chapter.

Supplementary prescribing

Supplementary prescribing arose from the 1999 Review of Prescribing, Supply and Administration of Medicines. The review suggested that appropriately trained non-medical health professionals, such as nurses and pharmacists, should be able to prescribe drugs within a Clinical Management Plan. The aim is to provide better and quicker patient care as well as to better use the skills of pharmacists and nurses. Their impact, however, is likely to be greatest in chronic diseases. Supplementary prescribing covers the general sales list, pharmacy-only medicines, prescription-only medicines and unlicensed medicines prescribed in certain instances. Controlled drugs were included in the list from April 2005.

Supplementary prescribing is a voluntary partnership between an independent prescriber – a physician or dentist – and a supplementary prescriber (SP), an appropriately trained pharmacist, or nurse. Management is defined in a common patient record and a Clinical Management Plan agreed between the independent prescriber (IP), supplementary prescriber and patient. Nevertheless, the stipulation that professionals must work within a Clinical Management Plan means that supplementary prescribing is likely to be most useful in chronic diseases, such as asthma, hypertension and diabetes mellitus. Initially, at least, nurses may be the most likely to benefit from the change. The infrastructure supporting nurse prescribing already exists. Furthermore, when possible, the DoH expects prescribing and dispensing to remain separate. This would minimise any potential concerns about probity.

Pharmacists

A pharmacist is an expert in drugs and medicines, who supplies medicines for the treatment or prevention of disease and can advise doctors and patients on their correct use. There are currently 16 schools of pharmacy and, from the summer of 2002, newly registered pharmacists will have passed through a four-year degree course to a 'Masters' level. The undergraduate teaching of pharmacists covers comprehensively the practical and theoretical knowledge of drugs and medicines. Once graduated a pre-registration year in practice (accredited by the Royal Pharmaceutical Society of Great Britain [RPSGB]) is completed. It is at this point that, after passing an exit exam, individuals are entered onto the Annual Register of Pharmaceutical Chemists.

Once registered, pharmacists occupy three main branches:

- community pharmacy
- hospital pharmacy
- the pharmaceutical industry.

The community pharmacist is generally the most frequent contact in primary care. However, we are also seeing the rise of a new branch of pharmacy, that being the practice-based pharmacist (see Chapter 9). As medicines management in primary care is deeply enshrined within the new contract, it offers an opportunity for doctors and pharmacists to work more closely together.

Pharmacist prescribing

The main route for pharmacist prescribing was originally via the supplementary prescribing scheme. Fully trained pharmacists wishing to become supplementary prescribers would have to undertake 25 taught days at an approved higher education institution, plus 12 days of learning in practice. These pharmacists too would require medical supervision and work within Clinical Management Plans. The 1 May 2006 changes to the regulations have enabled the creation of pharmacist independent prescribers. They too will be able to prescribe any licensed medicine within their level of competence and experience, though excluding all controlled drugs. In order to achieve this there will need to be some significant changes. Primarily, closer working relationships between GPs and community pharmacists will have to be forged. It is felt that primary care lags behind secondary care within this regard,[10] though many practices have excellent relationships with practice-based pharmacists (see Chapter 9). If the relationship between GPs and community pharmacists is pivotal, then there can be problems, as community pharmacies tend to have a mobile workforce, a large proportion working part time, and use locum pharmacists. Another potential problem may be pharmacists accessing patients' records. A pilot scheme overcame this via the use of electronic records and communication.[11] This may actually help accelerate GPs' transition from paper-based records, through paper-light to 'paperless' practice. This clearly has an IT resource implication. However, the 2005 Pharmacist New Contract creates an opportunity to encourage pharmacists as prescribers and fuel their evolution with plans of pharmacist independent prescribers in the future.

GPs may have concerns in relation to the commercial focus of the community pharmacist and the potential problems that could arise from that. However, an ethical study of community pharmacists who took on the prescribing of a general practice, for minor self-limiting illness, showed the costs stayed the same.[12] There would potentially be inequality, though, as GPs would have stricter regulations as to where and what they can dispense directly (see Chapter 7). Concerns may arise as to whether pharmacists can cope with the patient volume and yet maintain high standards. A barometer to the success of pharmacist prescribing will inevitably include the patient. However, this can be complicated by patients having clear views as to who does what,[13] rather than necessarily how well they do it. Despite this view, a pilot study of collaboration between GPs and pharmacists, for patients with coronary heart disease, showed this was possible.[14] Another successful national scheme has been for emergency hormonal contraception. Patients and doctors may well be sceptical and view supplementary prescribing as a second-rate, cost-cutting exercise. Doctors may consider this as competition and an erosion of their responsibilities, and it could fuel morale and recruitment difficulties. Plainly, it will require time, reassurance and education for doctors and patients to overcome this situation.

It is generally recognised that the NHS as a whole has developed good systems to support prescribers making cost-effective prescribing decisions. However, there is considerable avoidable waste and ill health. It is known that each year at least £100 million worth of medications is returned to pharmacists each year. Estimates of the number of hospital admissions that are due to problems with medicines range from 6 per cent to 10 per cent.[9] These figures, patient choice and government reform drive the supplementary prescribing process forwards.

To further aid pharmacist prescribing, it is envisaged that the range of over-the-counter medications will increase and make access to medicines easier for patients. Moreover, repeat dispensing by pharmacists, for patients requiring repeat medications, is in development. This will reduce the need for patients to visit their doctors for repeat prescriptions and allow pharmacists to closely monitor this area of prescribing (see Chapter 9).

In order for pharmacists and nurses to carry out supplementary prescribing there are some important procedural points that are worth noting. First, the doctor, nurse and pharmacist will all require access to a common patient record. Second, a confidential environment to consult will need to be available. This will be potentially particularly problematic for community pharmacists, where there would be a significant resource implication. However, despite the potential problems, supplementary prescribing can bring benefits to nurses and pharmacists, by way of role expansion.

For completeness, it is worth mentioning that dentists can also prescribe from a limited formulary. So, for example, dentists can prescribe some antibiotics for infections of the gum and teeth. However, dentists' responsibilities fall outside the scope of this book and interested readers would be advised to resource the relevant texts for further information.

When considering the introduction of new prescribers into primary care, it is worth looking further at some of the fundamentals that need to be in place. As always, the cornerstone to the success of this scheme will be adequate resources. This will require forward investment by the NHS and will not be a cheap alternative. Finally, any organisation is only as good as the people in it and this is no exception. Recruitment for mentors and pupils may be difficult as potential candidates look at the training, personal commitment and responsibility required. However, despite the bureaucracy, expanding the number of prescribing professionals will be an invaluable additional strategy for prescribing in primary care. It will allow us to utilise previously untapped resources and help primary care, working together, face the challenges ahead.

References

1. Moir D, Campbell H, Wrench J, *et al*. First steps in developing a Managed Clinical Network for vascular services in Lanarkshire. *Health Bull* 2001; **59**: 405–11.

2. Mughal MM, Mandell B, James K, *et al*. Implementing a shared-care approach to improve the management of patients with pulmonary arterial hypertension. *Cleve Clin J Med* 2003; **70** Supplement 1: S28–33.

3. Wagner G, Claes H, Costa P, *et al*. A shared care approach to the management of erectile dysfunction in the community. *Int J Impot Res* 2002; **14**: 189–94.

4. Dasgupta P, Drudge-Coates L, Smith K, *et al*. The cost effectiveness of a nurse-led shared-care prostate assessment clinic. *Ann R Coll Surg Engl* 2002; **84**: 328–30.

5. Curry R and Hollis J. An evolutionary approach to team working in primary care. *Br J Community Nurs* 2002; **7**: 520–7.

6. Withell B. A protocol for treating acute constipation in the community setting. *Br J Community Nurs* 2000; **5**: 110, 112, 114–17.

7. www.publications.doh.gov.uk/prescriptionstatistics/index.htm [accessed May 2006].

8. Warner TD and Mitchell JA. Cyclooxygenase-3 (COX-3): Filling in the gaps toward a COX continuum? *Proc Natl Acad Sci USA* 2002; **99**: 13371–3.

9. DoH. *Extending Independent Nurse Prescribing within the NHS in England: A Guide for Implementation*. London: DoH, March 2002.

10. Hughes C and McCann S. Perceived interprofessional barriers between community pharmacists and general practitioners: a qualitative assessment. *BJGP* 2003; **53**: 600–6.

11. Hassell K, Noyce PR, Rogers A, *et al*. Advice provided in British community pharmacies: What people want and what they get. *J Health Serv Res Policy* 1998; **3**; 219–25.

12. News Feature. Community pharmacist given direct access to GP records for reviews. *Pharm J* 2003: **270**; 787.

13. Petty D, Knapp P, Raynor DK, *et al*. Patients' views of a pharmacist-run medication review clinic in general practice. *BJGP* 2003; **53**: 607–13.

14. Ryan-Woolley BM and Cantrill J. Improving the care of community-based patients with ischaemic heart disease: A study of GP pharmacist collaboration, follow-up at one year. Report for St Helens & Knowsley HA and the DoH, 1999.

Annexe A

Controlled drugs that can be prescribed by Nurse Independent Prescribers (from 1 May 2006)

Substance	*Requirements as to use or route of administration*
Buprenorphine	Transdermal administration in palliative care
Chlordiazepoxide hydrochloride	Oral administration
Codeine phosphate	Oral administration
Co-phenotrope	Oral administration
Diamorphine hydrochloride	Oral or parenteral administration
Diazepam	Oral, parenteral or rectal administration
Dihydrocodeine tartrate	Oral administration
Fentanyl	Transdermal administration in palliative care
Lorazepam	Oral or parenteral administration
Midazolam	Parenteral or buccal administration
Morphine sulphate	Oral, parenteral or rectal administration
Morphine hydrochloride	Rectal administration
Oxycodone hydrochloride	Oral or parenteral administration in palliative care

Annexe B

Nurse Prescribers' Extended Formulary – list of medical conditions at February 2005

Circulatory
Haemorrhoids
Phlebitis – superficial

Ear
Furuncle
Otitis externa
Otitis media
Wax in ear

Endocrine
Hypoglycaemia

Eye
Blepharitis
Conjunctivitis, allergic
Conjunctivitis, infective
Local anaesthetic for ophthalmic conditions

Gastrointestinal conditions
Constipation
Gastroenteritis
Heartburn
Infantile colic
Worms – threadworms

Immunisations
Routine childhood and specific
  vaccinations

Musculoskeletal
Back pain – acute, uncomplicated
Neck pain – acute, uncomplicated
Soft tissue injury
Sprains

Annexe B continued

Oral conditions

Aphthous ulcer
Candidiasis, oral
Dental abscess
Gingivitis
Stomatitis

Respiratory

Acute attacks of asthma
Acute nasopharyngitis (coryza)
Laryngitis
Pharyngitis
Rhinitis, allergic
Sinusitis, acute
Tonsillitis

Skin

Abrasions
Acne
Animal and human bites
Boil/carbuncle
Burn/scald
Candidiasis, skin
Chronic skin ulcer
Dermatitis, atopic
Dermatitis, contact
Dermatitis, seborrhoeic
Dermatophytosis of the skin
(ringworm)
Herpes labialis
Impetigo
Insect bite/sting
Lacerations
Local anaesthetic for occasions when
   procedure requires it
Local anaesthetic for suturing of
lacerations
Nappy rash
Pediculosis (head lice)
Pruritus in chicken pox
Scabies

Urticaria
Warts (including verrucas)

Substance dependence

Smoking cessation

Urinary system

Urinary tract infection (women) –
   lower, uncomplicated

Female genital system

Bacterial vaginosis
Candidiasis, vulvovaginal
Contraception
Dysmenorrhoea
Emergency contraception
Laboratory-confirmed uncomplicated
   genital chlamydia infection (and the
   sexual partners of these patients)
Menopausal vaginal atrophy
Preconceptual counselling
Trichomonas vaginalis infection (and the
   sexual partners of these patients)

Male genital system

Balanitis

Palliative care

Anxiety
Bowel colic
Candidiasis, oral
Confusion
Constipation
Convulsions and restlessness
Cough
Dry mouth
Excessive respiratory secretions
Fungating malodorous tumours
Muscle spasm
Nausea and vomiting
Neuropathic pain in palliative care
Pain control

Chapter 5

The drive to prescribe

Colin Bradley

Introduction

Prescribing is a complex process with important technical, pharmacological, psychological, social, cultural, ethical and economic dimensions. Sometimes it is presented as simply a technical matter of applying the correct drug to the treatment of the correct disease, taking into consideration the patient's existing treatments and medical conditions. Even if tackled at this purely technical level prescribing can be a difficult and demanding task that requires considerable knowledge and skill on the part of the prescriber to get right. However, there are also the social and psychological dimensions of prescribing to be taken into account. Some researchers emphasise the potential clash of cultures between medical sciences. They tend to focus on the technical aspects of prescribing and the culture of patients, who can be sceptical of the claims of medicinal science and who may be more focused on wishes, desires and their so called 'lived experience'. It is sometimes even implied that the technical, rational world of medicine is incompatible with the life world of patients' actual experience and that the demands of one can only be met at the cost of frustrating the demands of the other. However, this is not necessarily the case and the real challenge in prescribing is to marry the different aspects in a way that is technically competent, psycho-socially sensitive, ethically sound and economically responsible.

The prescribing process

Prescribing is a process and not a single event or act (see Figure 5.1). The process can be said to begin when the patient who is ill, or believes himself or herself to be ill, consults a doctor with a view to receiving a treatment to make them well again. The doctor, traditionally, but now the prescriber (of whatever hue) undertakes a process of ascertaining the nature of the patient's problem or problems. On the basis of this assessment the prescriber may decide what, if anything, ails the patient and on the basis of this assessment will usually select an appropriate treatment or treatments. It is increasingly argued that patients often can and usually should be actively involved in the process of deciding the nature of the problem(s) and in selecting the most appropriate treatment. A treatment, having been selected, will then, typically, be written on a prescription to be dispensed by a pharmacist. The prescription comprises a set of instructions to the pharmacist regarding what drug or drugs are to be dispensed, the form in which they are to be dispensed, the quantity to be dispensed and the manner in which they are to be taken by the patient. The pharmacist is usually relied upon to convey to the patient the dosing frequency and regimen and duration of treatment (see Chapter 6). After the prescription has been written and dispensed there is a process by which the patient consumes the medicine (or perhaps fails to consume the medicine), which may or may not correspond to the instructions given by either doctor or pharmacist or, ideally, both. The process of prescribing also includes the sharing of information about the condition(s) and the drug(s) with the patient, and information about whether or not the medicine has the desired effect(s) and any undesired effect(s). Thus prescribing is a long process that involves many parties including at a minimum a doctor (or other prescriber), a pharmacist (or other supplier of the medicine(s)) and the patient.

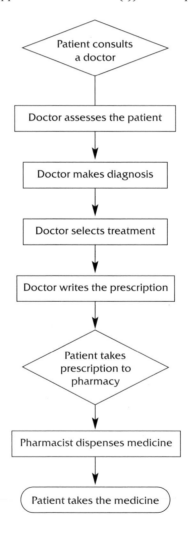

Figure 5.1: Traditional view of the prescribing process

The consultation

The prescribing process, usually, begins with a consultation between doctor (most commonly) and patient. At its simplest the consultation consists of a patient telling the doctor their complaint. The doctor asks questions and, perhaps, examines the patient, and on the basis of the information obtained deduces the diagnosis of the patient's condition. On the basis of this conclusion the doctor selects an appropriate remedy, which they then prescribe for the patient. Ideally, the patient takes this and gets better. However, this description of the consultation is much too simplistic and what is actually occurring is considerably more complex. First, consultations are not always concerned with a new condition presenting in the patient for the first time. Many consultations are about existing or recurring problems; they may concern not just one but several problems. In general practice they typically occur in the context of a series of consultations between doctor and patient where mutual learning about each other has already occurred. This has a direct influence on what happens in any given consultation. Furthermore, the patient is not usually anything like as passive a participant in the consultation process as the initial description given above would suggest.

Even where the patient is consulting for the first time with a new complaint, perhaps even to a previously unknown doctor, there may be many factors already at play that will have a strong bearing on the outcome of the consultation. The patient will usually have thought a good deal about the symptoms that will have brought them to the doctor. They will have interpreted these symptoms in the light of any previous experience of these or similar symptoms and their prior knowledge of possible disease causes and the treatment they might require. Patients may even have tried to wait to see if the problem resolves spontaneously, or they may have tried some home remedies or some over-the-counter medications (OTC). They will most probably have sought advice from others in their family or circle of friends. From previous experience with illness and with doctors in general, they will be able to anticipate the kinds of things the doctor might say or do and they may well have expectations regarding how their complaint should be handled. New presentations of symptoms to a doctor are most typically provoked by a degree of anxiety about the possible significance of the symptoms, but they may be provoked by a perceived need to access particular treatments such as antibiotics, which can only be accessed by prescription in the United Kingdom. Sometimes the decision to consult may be driven by the need for validation of the illness by means of a doctor's certificate, for example, and may not involve any prescribing issues at all.

Patients with more chronic health problems have different needs. They may have less need for a diagnosis, although if there has been a change in their chronic illness they may need some explanation for this. They may need the management of their condition reviewed and this may involve routine laboratory tests and so forth. The patient may have more complex and subliminal needs to have their suffering recognised and acknowledged, to get help with adapting to their illness and the sense of loss it induces. They may simply need to share with their doctor their experiences of living with their illness as someone whose specialist knowledge, they hope, will incline them to show a greater understanding of their experience than, perhaps, other people they interact with. Sometimes patients need help in understanding their illness and how it affects them, as well as gaining knowledge about its treatment. They may also need assistance in identifying and deciding on how to respond to undesirable effects of their treatment. They need an explanation of the risks of their illness, such as complications and advice on how they can contain these risks.

Given this variation in the nature and content of consultations, the requirements of the prescribing element will vary from consultation to consultation. It may be that a prescription is not required. This may raise patient concerns as to why a prescription is not being issued, or regarding drugs prescribed on previous occasions. There are, however, some key elements of how prescribing is performed within the consultation that are common to virtually all types of consultation. First, prescribing involves weighing up risks and benefits of treatments, and this requires adequate knowledge of the probabilities associated with these risks and benefits. Second, the prescribing process involves the sharing of a considerable body of information in most instances and the prescriber requires high levels of communication skills to successfully manage this information exchange. Third, it is increasingly recognised that patients may have important and valid views on what is to be prescribed, and these views should be sought and taken into account. However, it is also acknowledged that, while patients invariably have a view on their treatment, they do not always want to share this view and they vary in the extent to which they want to be actively involved in the decision making. While it is generally good practice and ethically desirable that patients should be involved in treatment decisions, this should not be forced on patients who are unwilling or unable to participate.

These insights should translate into an approach to the consultation which begins from a recognition that consultations take place within the context of a doctor–patient relationship and that this relationship should, where possible, be enhanced by the process of any individual consultation (see Figure 5.2). This means that prescribers should begin by trying to see the problem from the patient's perspective. This requires recognition of and sensitivity to the patient's ideas, concerns and expectations as well as how it affects them physically, psychologically and socially.[1] These thoughts may be formed by a wide variety of influences to which the doctor should also be alert, including the patient's religious and cultural background, their emotional state and their prior experiences of illness and medical care. Having obtained, from the patient, a clear view of the problem(s) from their perspective, the doctor's first task is to determine whether the symptoms presented represent, or are likely to represent, an identifiable disease. If this is the case the doctor's next task will be to put a label (or diagnosis) on the problem(s) and reach a shared understanding with the patient of the problem(s), any investigations necessary and treatments available. One needs to recognise that patients will vary in the extent to which they are able to absorb the information that is given in a consultation. This perhaps can be improved by the use of patient information leaflets,[2] though this previously accepted tool has been recently challenged.[3] It is also well recognised that patients vary in the extent to which they want to be involved in prescribing decisions. However, the clearer the prescriber is in their explanations and instructions the more likely it is the patient will be able to absorb the information. Likewise, with appropriate skills in communicating risks and benefits, the easier it will be for patients to participate realistically in the decision-making process.[4]

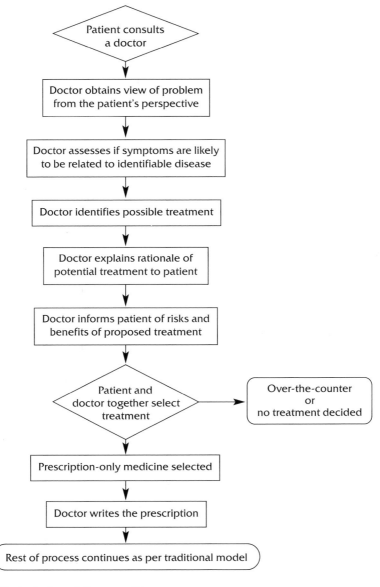

Figure 5.2: Revised view of the prescribing process

A good many problems that present in primary care are benign and self-limiting, and may be capable of management by the patient themselves using simple home remedies or over-the-counter treatments. Where this applies there is a strong case for encouraging the patient to manage the problem without recourse to prescription medicines, mainly because to encourage and guide such self-management empowers the patient and makes them more capable of and confident in managing their own health in the future. It may also be financially advantageous too if they are liable for prescription charges. Exemption from prescription charges may create a somewhat stronger case for prescribing medicines, even if they are available over the counter. Indeed, this may be the sole reason for the consultation.

Effective prescribing

The doctor's goal is to prescribe effectively, which means balancing the needs and desires of the patient with considerations of safety, efficacy and economy. Effective prescribing can be said to incorporate the following elements:

- diagnosis of the patient's condition, usually on history and examination but including the appropriate use of investigations
- selecting appropriate treatment from the range of possible options with due consideration of non-drug options and in the light of pre-existing illnesses and possible drug–drug interactions
- tailoring the treatment to the patient
- setting up appropriate monitoring arrangements to monitor the course of the illness, the response to treatment and to detect the emergence of any adverse effects.

Diagnosis

Ideally, prescribing should be driven by diagnosis. In general practice, however, complete and accurate diagnosis is not always achievable. This arises for a number of reasons. Patients in general practice present with symptoms rather than with diseases. Symptoms may be indicative of normal physiology, e.g. palpitations associated with anxiety; they may be indicative of known disease and not require any new therapeutic response; they may be indicative of self-limiting illness that will resolve with or without treatment; and they may be indicative of new illness with potentially serious and longer-term consequences. Sorting these is a major task for general practice. A thorough history with an appropriate focus on the most probable explanations but with a weather eye to the more sinister if remote possibilities is the essence of the required approach. Thus, for example, an adult presenting with a cough has most probably got a cold but one needs to bear in mind the possibilities of pneumonia, bronchitis (chronic or acute) and, especially if elderly or a smoker, lung cancer. Time is used as an important diagnostic tool, with a judicious wait often allowing one to retrospectively recognise the benign and short-lived cause of the symptoms while saving the patient and the health service the expense, inconvenience and possible hazards of investigations. However, GPs will often recognise what might be called 'red flag' symptoms that prompt a more vigorous response on initial presentation and lead to earlier investigation and more specific treatment. For instance, in the example above, the presence of wheeze, in addition, might prompt a more detailed history and examination for possible asthma that, if found to be likely, would indicate treatment with bronchodilators and possibly inhaled corticosteroids. Likewise, the finding of recent weight loss and/or anaemia might prompt more urgent investigation of the possibility of lung cancer.

As well as presenting mainly with symptoms, patients in general practice, even those with what ultimately prove to be significant illnesses, rarely have clear-cut signs. This is because in primary care diseases are often seen at an early stage in their development when symptoms may be apparent but signs have not yet developed. Furthermore, patients may present with a mixture of symptoms some of which are related to their primary problem and others which are not. Often these latter are symptoms of the co-existing anxiety that accompanies most patients' initial presentations to doctors. Patients may also have a mixture of relevant and irrelevant (or coincidental) signs. Patients can present with signs in the absence of symptoms and with symptoms that do not fit with any pattern of known illness. All in all, the capacity of patient presentations in general practice to baffle their doctors is enormous. However, fortunately, most presentations of symptoms and signs do fit recognisable patterns and doctors must recognise these in order to achieve the best possible diagnosis.

The role of investigations in making diagnoses is not always well understood. Occasionally, a diagnosis will be made mainly or exclusively on the basis of a test. However, the role of investigations is in either ruling in or ruling out a particular diagnosis or range of diagnoses. It is in the authors' opinion that 80–90 per cent of diagnoses are made on the history alone, with examination adding another few per cent and laboratory tests adding very little. The role of laboratory testing, therefore, is more often to firm up and/or clarify a diagnosis that has already suggested itself from the history and examination. Thus, in the above example, a normal full blood count (FBC) would help rule out anaemia as a cause of breathlessness, whereas an abnormal FBC might suggest that cancer is more likely. A chest X-ray would, likewise, be used to confirm a clinical diagnosis of pneumonia (were such a diagnosis to have been made clinically). Another major role of laboratory tests is in the monitoring of the continuing course of an illness and in detecting the beneficial and/or adverse effects of medicines, of which more below.

Selecting appropriate treatment

An accurate diagnosis is the key to selecting a specific and appropriate treatment, although, as noted above, this is not always achievable. Where a reasonably accurate diagnosis can be made there will still usually be a range of treatments to choose from. Many problems presenting in general practice will resolve regardless of treatment and, in these instances, the goal is to select a treatment that will provide adequate symptom relief to the patient while minimising costs and risks of the treatment. For many such problems a non-drug treatment may be appropriate and may even be sufficient on its own. Again, in the cough example, honey and lemon drinks and steam inhalations are as likely to be helpful as any cough mixture.[5] Antipyretics may also be useful. These, though, can usually be purchased over the counter and this approach should generally be encouraged rather than prescribing them, as this helps the patient to take the management of their illness into their own hands where this is appropriate. The aim in the management of such minor ailments should generally be to put treatment into the hands of the patient. Thus empowering patients will enable them to manage such conditions themselves. The time spent educating patients is time well spent, as it will increase patient satisfaction and reduce future consultations for similar conditions.

When it comes to selecting treatment for more serious health problems, the prescriber needs to balance safety, efficacy, suitability for the patient and cost. In a primary care setting where the stage a disease manifests may well be earlier and the probability of serious disease is less, it may be argued that safety ought to be the higher priority. In hospital, by contrast, the greater inherent risks of the disease may justify the placing of a higher priority on efficacy. All drugs carry a risk of adverse effects, which may be predictable from characteristics of the patient, the dose and regimen used. However, some adverse effects are intrinsically unpredictable (idiosyncratic). Predictable side effects can often be avoided, though vigilance is needed by both the patient and prescriber with regard to idiosyncratic adverse effects. Predictable risks include the known greater risk in elderly patients to adverse drug effects, mainly related to declining renal and/or hepatic function (covered in detail in Chapter 9). Children, too, may handle drugs differently and doses generally need to be adjusted to allow for both lower body weight (or body surface area) and differences in drug handling. Therefore, drug selection should take account of existing conditions the patient is known to have and the patient's age.

Regardless of whether or not co-existing conditions make a difference to which drugs can be safely prescribed, the treatment of other conditions with drugs also poses risks when new drugs come to be added. The use of multiple drugs in the same patient is known to pose risks associated with interactions between drugs. These, too, may be predictable from known qualities and effects of each drug, but they can also be unpredictable. They are possibly related to genetically determined differences in the extent and speed with which different people metabolise different medicines. Prescribers used to be urged to be generally cautious about the risks of 'polypharmacy', defined sometimes as more than one, more than three, or more than four drugs simultaneously taken by the same patient. It is increasingly recognised, however, that certain combinations of treatments have a high probability of generating clinical problems due to their interaction,[6] while other combinations have little or no probability of interactions. Furthermore, with developments in preventive medicine it is often seen that, while single treatments reduce some risks by a given amount, combinations of treatments are needed to lower risk to the maximum extent possible. Usually, the combinations recommended are known not to interact or to interact in ways that are, overall, of benefit to the patient. An example of this may be a hypertensive patient who requires lifestyle changes, antihypertensives, a lipid-lowering agent and aspirin. Thus, if polypharmacy is defined purely in terms of the number of agents a patient is on simultaneously we would have to elaborate on this to distinguish between 'good polypharmacy', where the patient is on combinations of drugs that have been shown to be safe and effective, and 'bad' or 'undesirable polypharmacy', where the combination is likely to be more harmful than beneficial.

While safety is of paramount concern, the drugs prescribed for patients need to be effective as well. For many conditions and symptoms there is a range of effective treatments available. Sometimes these will be drugs in the same therapeutic class with broadly similar pharmacological properties and little between them in terms of efficacy. Potency (see Chapter 2) may vary a lot between drugs of the same pharmacological class but this should not usually be an issue in the selection of drugs if the effect achieved is similar. Where drugs are of similar efficacy the choice of drug will be made on other grounds, such as side effect profile or cost. Sometimes, there may be real differences in efficacy between drugs available to treat a particular condition and it is important to choose the most effective one. This might be capable of being determined on the basis of therapeutic studies undertaken and reported in the research literature. Well-designed therapeutic trials will generate a figure for number needed to treat (NNT) and the lower this figure the more efficacious the treatment. However, efficacy can vary from patient to patient for the same drug and one may have to determine by a process of trial and error what works for a particular patient. For example, there is a range of drug classes available for the treatment of hypertension. The precise effect on a given patient's blood pressure by a drug of a particular class can be quite unpredictable. Diuretics and beta-blockers are first choice for the treatment of hypertension as stated in NICE guidelines[7] not because they are more efficacious than other classes of drugs but because they are effective, cheap and, generally speaking, equally safe (the author notes that the British Hypertension Society guidelines[8] offer a different view and interested readers are directed towards the relevant reference). Blood pressure may require treatment with several different antihypertensive drugs before the required target level for that patient is found.

Tailoring the treatment to the patient

Finding the drug with the greatest effect for the patient is only one aspect of tailoring the treatment to the patient. This phrase more usually refers to selecting the medicine that best suits the patient from the formulations available, or to adjusting the dosing regimen to match the patient's lifestyle. For instance, diuretics are usually given in the morning so that the patient will be up and about, and be easily able to get to the toilet. However, for elderly patients who have arthritis, mobility may be more restricted first thing in the morning and getting to the toilet is easier as the day wears on. In this case administering the diuretic slightly later in the day is a form or tailoring the regimen to the patient. The prescriptions of syrups for children and soluble forms of medicine for people who have difficulties swallowing are other examples of tailoring the medicine to the patient. Likewise, the choice of inhaler technology – dry-powder versus metered-dose inhaler – may well be something that is chosen to meet patients' requirements. All these measures will improve patient concordance.

Appropriate monitoring arrangements

Patients on long-term therapies generally need to be monitored. First, they need to be monitored to determine whether the medicine is having the expected effects. Second, they need to be monitored to ensure the medicine is not causing any adverse effects. Finally, they may need to be monitored for any possible deterioration of their condition that might prompt a reconsideration of their treatment. In many long-term conditions there are known markers of the degree of disease control being achieved. For example, in diabetes, HbA1c is a good marker of glycaemic control. In hypertension, blood pressure is an obvious indicator. In asthma, peak flow is one measure but history of nocturnal symptoms is another good indicator of degree of control. For other treatments it is the potential adverse effects that require regular monitoring. For example, patients on methotrexate need regular full blood counts to detect the possible development of aplastic anaemia. In a minority of instances, for example in anti-epilepsy treatment, there may be methods for monitoring drug concentration in the patient's blood. However, therapeutic blood monitoring needs to be used judiciously. It can be quite expensive and, unless the result is likely to lead to some significant change in treatment, it may not be worthwhile for either the doctor or patient.

Besides being aware of what needs to be monitored for and how often monitoring is required, prescribers need to establish robust management systems to ensure that required monitoring happens when it should. As the medicines that require monitoring tend to be long term, and prescriptions for long-term medications tend to be issued as repeat prescriptions, these systems amount to repeat prescribing systems. An academic pharmacist named Zermansky[9] has pointed out that an effective repeat prescribing system has three components, namely a front-office (day-to-day or tactical) management system, a back-office (or strategic) management system and a clinical management system. Safe and cost-effective repeat prescribing requires attention to all these aspects. Thus the front-office management system is where the request for the repeat prescription is received. There needs to be a robust system to ensure every request gets picked up, logged, and the wheels set in motion for the prescription to be written and issued. The front-office system also needs to check if the patient is, in fact, authorised for the repeat prescription requested and then ensure that it is recorded when the prescription is handed over to the patient or their representative. The back-office system has to determine how requests are dealt with once they are received. There need to be policies on: how long the turnaround should normally be; what information is needed by the doctor before signing the prescription; what is to be done with urgent requests, requests that are out of synchronisation with expected repeat intervals and so on. The clinical management system deals with matters such as: what needs to be monitored when a repeat prescription request is made; how often the patient should be seen; what is to be checked when they are seen; and how to deal with requests that are made prematurely or belatedly. These latter two issues relate to the issue of adherence or compliance. Requests being made too early suggest the patient is taking the medicine too frequently – sometimes called 'over-compliance' – whereas requests being made too late suggest 'under-compliance'. The face-to-face review that should occur at regular intervals is sometimes called a 'therapeutic review'. It should include: a review of symptoms of the illness or illnesses that lead to the repeat prescription; a review of the patient's perception of the benefits of the medication; a review of any possible adverse effects of the medicine(s) being experienced by the patient; and a general review of the patient's general health to detect any other health problems emerging.

Prescribing in context

Prescribing does not occur in isolation between doctor and patient. Rather it occurs in a wider context including the context of the patient's and the doctor's prior knowledge and experience; in the context of the information available to the doctor and, increasingly, the patient; in the context of the primary healthcare team; and in the context of the NHS.

Doctors' knowledge and experience

Doctors, in common with all human decision makers, have to make their decisions within the limits of the information available to them. Given the substantial role prescribing plays in general practice it is appropriate that GPs' knowledge of medicines should be quite substantial. However, considering the enormous diversity of the potential range of problems that can present and the ever-expanding range of drugs available, it is not reasonable to expect every GP to know everything that could possibly be relevant to the pharmaceutical care of every patient they might see. This requires that doctors also have a knowledge acquisition and utilisation strategy. That is to say, doctors need to have a reasonably comprehensive knowledge of a smallish range of drugs they use regularly. They also need a readily available source of sufficient and reliable information on drugs they might have to use when encountering a patient whose problem lies outside the range of what is commonly dealt with. There have been a number of attempts to define a minimal set of drugs that would deal effectively with 90 per cent or so of problems presenting in primary care. The World Health Organization (WHO) essential drug list,[10] although advanced originally for the developing world, is one such list. Various practice formularies that have been proposed over the years are others. Such lists tend to contain in the order of 200 or so medicines that are said to be capable of treating 90 per cent or more of problems presenting to GPs. In relation to this list the prescriber could be reasonably expected to have a good working knowledge of the indications for the drug, the potential adverse effects, the contraindications, the important interactions, usual doses and dosing regimen, and durations of treatment, i.e. they should know enough to be able to prescribe the drug safely and effectively. Furthermore, they should have some idea on how the drug is handled (i.e. metabolised, distributed and excreted) in the body and what dose adjustments or other precautions, if any, are needed in the treatment of older patients and others with impairments of drug handling. The prescriber, ideally, ought to have an idea of the drug's cost or at least cost relative to alternative drugs for the same purpose. He or she also needs to know the drug's legal status, particularly if it is a controlled drug, and any special prescribing requirements or restrictions.

Prescribers need to know and understand some more general aspects of prescribing practice such as how, broadly, drugs are licensed and how their safety is assured (see Chapter 3). Doctors need to be aware, for instance, of the requirements on them to report adverse drug reactions using the 'Yellow Card' reporting system (see Chapter 9). Doctors need to appreciate the public health and economic implications of prescribing. They need to be aware of the societal issue of drug misuse and how they can contribute to its containment through judicious prescribing of drugs of potential misuse. They should subscribe to the concept of evidence-based medicine and pursue opportunities to keep their knowledge up-to-date and in line with best evidence.

What distinguishes doctors skilled in their craft from relative novices is often not so much their greater knowledge but their greater experience. One product of experience is that one organises and uses one's knowledge more effectively rather than necessarily having more knowledge. GPs' experience is not just of the presentations of illness and the effects of medicines on illness, but of people in general and their attitudes, motivations and behaviours. GPs also build up a fund of knowledge of particular people, which enables them to be better prescribers. This makes up part of the process of 'life long learning'.

Patients' knowledge and experience

Patients, too, come to a consultation with their own body of knowledge and experience. They may have previous experience with the particular symptoms or condition they are consulting with and they will have experience of illness in general. They will have some prior experience of drugs including, possibly, drugs used for their current symptoms. They also generally have prior experiences with doctors in general and, often, with the particular GP they are consulting. All these prior experiences influence what happens during any given consultation. This applies whether or not a prescription is issued and always whether or not any drug prescribed is actually taken. Patients have their own body of knowledge of diseases and possibly of their own disease too, especially if they have had the disease for some time or the disease is one that has been experienced by others of their close acquaintance. The information and understanding they have may or may not concur with the prevailing medical view. Likewise, patients have their own knowledge base of medicines both in general and in particular, which, again, may be more or less congruent with the medical view. Increasingly, patients are getting more and more access to information about diseases and medicines through all media but, perhaps, most particularly through the internet. The quality and reliability of this information varies greatly and patients do not always have the wherewithal to make judgements on the information they access. In the information age the role of the prescriber, for some patients at least, is shifting from being a source of knowledge and directive advice to that of interpreter of information and a guide to patients making their own choices.

Information available

As noted above, doctors need to have a good knowledge of a small repertoire of drugs they use regularly. However, they must also recognise the need to appreciate the limitations of that knowledge and have an understanding of where to seek further appropriate and reliable information when their own resource is exceeded. GPs in the UK are fortunate in having ready access to a number of very good sources of such information. The traditional linchpin of prescribing information has been the *British National Formulary*, which provides a good balance between comprehensive coverage and manageable size, such that it can be kept on a desk, in a bag or wherever one is seeing patients. It is now available on the internet.[11] This source is supplemented by the *Drug and Therapeutics Bulletin*, which provides independent reviews of therapeutic issues. These draw attention to key issues in medicines use, including how and when to use particular drugs. Others such as the *MeReC Bulletin* follow the same format but place an emphasis on other issues determined by their originators, such as economics and cost-effectiveness in prescribing. These sources are now complemented by information derived from the evidence-based medicine enterprise such as the *Cochrane Database* and *Clinical Evidence* (published by the *British Medical Journal* publishing group). They are available electronically (free of charge in the UK) to all prescribers.

Detailed knowledge of individual drugs, however, is only a starting point for good prescribing. Prescribers also need guidance on when different drugs available for the treatment of the same condition are put to best use. Prescribers may also need guidance on how to evaluate the clinical problem prior to any prescribing decision and they may need guidance on monitoring and other aspects of management in addition to drug information. Such information is increasingly available in the evidence base but not always in a form that is easy to implement. Thus, the research evidence is more and more being consolidated into the form of guidelines that aim to deal with all the common issues that arise in the diagnosis and management of most clinical problems. Guidelines, like other information sources to guide treatment, vary in their quality and the extent to which they are evidence based, so it behoves prescribers to learn how to distinguish creditable and practical guidelines from less valuable ones and learn how to apply appropriate ones. It must also be stressed that guidelines are only just for guidance and there will also always be a need for clinicians to exercise judgement, particularly with regard to when it is appropriate to go beyond the guidelines.

A step on from written guidelines are information and decision support systems that aim to bring the information from guidelines and other evidence-based sources directly into the process of prescribing in real time. An example of such a system is PRODIGY,[12] which is a decision support tool. This can be integrated into the practice's clinical record system so that, as the prescriber is recording clinical data, relevant diagnostic and therapeutic information is supplied to support and guide both diagnostic and therapeutic decisions. Thus, for example, if one records 'cough' as a symptom the system may, if required, suggest a range of probable diagnoses. If one selects 'asthma' as the diagnosis the system may then suggest treatments based on guidelines such as the British Thoracic Society Guidelines.[13]

Primary healthcare team

Historically, prescribing largely occurred in the context of a relationship and consultations between individual doctors and patients. This is no longer the case. GPs now work in primary healthcare teams with other health professionals, several of whom are now also able to prescribe for the patient. Furthermore, other members of the team – particularly pharmacists – are available to inform and advise the GP on their prescribing practice. In the past, prescribing decisions – including decisions of whether or not to prescribe, what to prescribe and whether or not to prescribe a new drug or cease using an old drug – were taken by the GP alone, often within the course of individual consultations. It is now recognised that decisions do not all have to be made in the heat of the consultation, as it were. Many decisions can be made, at least provisionally, in anticipation of certain situations arising in practice. Thus, for example, decisions about which antibiotic to use for commonly encountered infections can be made in the context of developing a practice formulary or drawing up local guidelines. Then when the question of which antibiotic is required arises with a patient the doctor can draw on the prior decisions made. A major advantage of this approach – of discussing treatments prior to a situation arising – is that other team members can contribute to the decision from their own expertise. A further advantage is that different prescribers working together will behave consistently with regards patients, which will tend to discourage the patients making inappropriate requests. Other team members without specific expertise in therapeutics provide other treatment modalities that may be alternatives to prescribing or may be adjuncts to drug treatments.

NHS context

Being a healthcare system striving to provide comprehensive care to the entire population, and funded almost entirely by taxes, the NHS has the capacity and motivation to regulate a good deal of the prescribing environment. Thus there are government-determined policies, regulations and sometimes laws supervising virtually every aspect of prescribing. While individual clinical decisions are not dictated by legislation or regulation there are increasingly sophisticated attempts to influence or guide the prescribing of clinicians in ways that meet government objectives for prescribing. The government has two principal objectives in exercising its influence on prescribing. On the one hand, there is the self-evident desire to get the best health care it can and, on the other, there is the desire to do so at the minimum cost. On the supply side there are government influences on the pharmaceutical industry such as the Pharmaceutical Price Regulation Scheme – an agreement between the industry and the government that limits overall prices paid by the NHS for pharmaceuticals. The government also has agreements with pharmacists that are also designed to limit costs, such as the agreement that when a prescription is written generically the pharmacist will only be reimbursed at a level set in the Drug Tariff,[14] which is typically at or about the price of the cheapest generic brand available. Thus, if the pharmacist supplies a more expensive brand they take a potential reduction in profit. Also if pharmacists negotiate discounts there are arrangements whereby the government shares in the benefits of such discounts too (see Chapter 7).

On the demand side there are various government policies and directives that are designed to both reduce costs and maximise the value obtained from prescribing expenditure. These include such initiatives as: National Service Frameworks, which offer guidance on the optimum management of clinical problems that may often encourage prescribing where it is deemed to be associated with sufficient health gain; NICE guidance, which is concerned with distinguishing treatments that offer good value for money from those deemed to offer poor value for money; and prescribing budgets, which are more explicitly directed at minimising expenditure on medicines albeit providing this is not at the expense of patient care. More recent developments include the establishment of Primary Care Trusts with overall responsibility for all prescribing expenditure, and the introduction of more formalised clinical governance and developments in IT, which reinforce and bring a new level of sophistication to these efforts to maximise the cost-effectiveness of primary care prescribing expenditure. While it has always been the case that prescribers have been under some obligation to take into consideration the overall context of the NHS, this inescapable fact of life is coming to be more explicitly operationalised in individual consultations through recent policy initiatives. Other policy initiatives, such as the new GP contract, while not so directly concerned with prescribing *per se* will further enhance the implementation of these prescribing directives.

Having, in the past, concerned themselves almost exclusively with the efficacy and costs of medicines the government and various health agencies are now also beginning to turn their attention to safety of medicines use. The National Patient Safety Agency (NPSA) and others have begun to examine the area of medication error and how to avoid what is now referred to as 'preventable drug-related morbidity' (PDRM). This area is covered more fully in the chapters to come.

References

1. O'Gara PE and Fairhurst W. Therapeutic communication: General approaches that enhance the quality of the consultation. *Accident and Emergency Nursing* 2004; **12(3)**: 166–72.
2. Kenny T, Wilson R and Purves IR. Prescribing Patient Information Leaflets may be better than drugs. *BMJ* 1998; **317(7150)**: 80–1.
3. Clarke Moloney M, Moore A, Adelola OA, *et al*. Information leaflets for venous leg ulcer patients: Are they effective? *Br J Wound Care* 2005; **14(2)**: 75–7.
4. McCormack JP, Dolovich L, Levine M, *et al*. Providing evidence based information to patients and pharmacies: What is the acceptability, usefulness and impact? *Health Expect* 2003; **6(4)**: 281–9.
5. Editorial: Complex choices tackling common cold. *Pharma J* 2004; **272**: 34.
6. Fulton M and Riley AE. Polypharmacy in the elderly. A literature review. *J Am Acad Nurse Pract* 2005; **17(4)**: 123–32.
7. National Institute for Health and Clinical Excellence. www.nice.org.uk [accessed May 2006].
8. www.bhsoc.org/Latest_BHS_management_Guidelines.htm [accessed May 2006].
9. Zermansky AG. Clinical medication review by a pharmacist of patients on repeat prescriptions in general practice. *Health Technol Assess* 2002; **6(20)**: 1–86.
10. World Health Organization essential drug list. www.who.int/mediacentre/factsheets [accessed May 2006].
11. *British National Formulary*. www.bnf.org/bnf/.
12. PRODIGY. www.prodigy.nhs.uk [accessed May 2006].
13. British Thoracic Society Guidelines. www.brit-thoracic.org.uk/iqs/sid.0113394032162384 2708480/Guidelinessince%201997_asthma_html [accessed May 2006].
14. The Drug Tariff. www.ppa.org.uk/edt/May_2005/mindex.htm [accessed May 2006].

Chapter 6

Writing a prescription

Brian Crichton

The writing of a prescription punctuates a vital stage in the management of a patient. It enables patients to obtain the medicines that their prescriber plans, in the form, dosage and amount required. To achieve this, the prescriber needs a detailed understanding of the rules and regulations for writing a prescription and be able to avoid the potential pitfalls. This chapter will help equip the reader with the knowledge required to achieve this.

In 2002, 650 million prescriptions were dispensed in England, i.e. 12.4 scripts per head of the population.[1] Despite this fact, our patients have access to a huge array of over-the-counter (OTC) medicines that can be useful for many ailments. In addition there are many drugs that are available as prescription-only medicines (POM). The number and types of POM vary from country to country and a complete list of these drugs, for the United Kingdom, can be found in the *British National Formulary* (BNF).[2]

The terms of service for doctors state that (subject to paragraph 39 and 41 to 44)

> a prescriber shall order any drugs, medicines or appliances which are needed for the treatment of any patient who is receiving treatment under the contract by issuing to that patient a prescription form or a repeatable prescription and such a prescription form or repeatable prescription shall not be used in any other circumstances.[3]

This means that a GP can't use the FP10 form to prescribe swimming sessions, yoga, etc. However, a doctor can prescribe any drug or appliance as an NHS pharmaceutical service. There has to be limitations on what can be prescribed at NHS expense and it is important that prescribers only prescribe within their own competencies. These limitations lie within Paragraph 42 of the General Medical Services (GMS) Contract[3] and take two main forms. First, there are the drugs not listed in the Drug Tariff that are called Schedule 1 drugs in the GP GMS Contract (previously called Schedule 10, the 'Black List') and, second, those on Schedule 2 (previously called Schedule 11, the 'Selected List'). Schedule 1 drugs are not prescribable under the NHS and a complete list can be found in the NHS GMS's regulations[3] and section 18b of the Drug Tariff (see Chapter 7). An example is that of oil of evening primrose, which has recently been classified into this schedule. With regard to Schedule 2, these Selected List

Table 6.1: Criteria for Schedule 2 prescribing in erectile dysfunction under the NHS	
Diabetes mellitus	Severe pelvic injury
Multiple sclerosis	Single-gene neurological disease
Spina bifida	Parkinson's disease
Spinal cord injury	Poliomyelitis
Carcinoma of the prostate	
A man who is receiving treatment for renal failure by dialysis	
A man who has severe psychological sequelae caused by his erectile dysfunction	
A man who has had the following surgery: • prostatectomy • radical pelvic surgery • renal failure treated by transplant	

Scheme (SLS) drugs within the Drug Tariff are titled 'Part XVIIIB – Drugs to be prescribed in certain circumstances under the NHS Pharmaceutical Services'. SLS endorsement on the Rx is a requirement for the medicinal product to be allowed on the NHS (see below under prescription endorsements). An example of a group of drugs in this section would be those prescribed in erectile dysfunction. Table 6.1 lists the conditions where these particular drugs can be prescribed through the NHS.

If an individual does not fall within these set criteria, then they are not entitled to an NHS prescription for that condition. Sometimes certain foods and toilet preparations can be regarded as drugs and the Advisory Committee on Borderline Substances (ACBS) states in what circumstances this can occur. A list of such substances and the conditions deemed applicable by the ACBS can be found in the BNF and Drug Tariff.

For other prescribers (see Chapter 4) there are formularies that fulfil their individual prescribing needs, e.g. the Dental Practitioners' and Nurse Prescribers' Formularies. These contain a smaller number of drugs that have been approved by the secretary of state and can be found listed in the BNF.

The method through which we make a written request to a pharmacist to supply a medication for a patient is via a prescription. It is to this that we can now turn our attention.

Types of prescription

There are basically two main types of prescription. First, there are the standard NHS FP10 prescriptions. These are the most common types of prescription issued in the

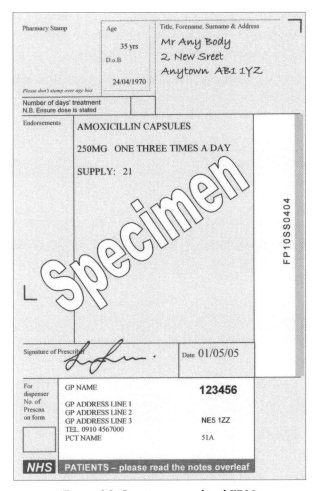

Figure 6.1: Specimen completed FP10

United Kingdom and can be handwritten or computer generated, with both having the same standard format (see Figure 6.1). Second, there are private prescriptions. These are non-NHS prescriptions and are not regulated in the same way as NHS prescriptions. To gain a greater understanding of the different types of prescription, a fuller consideration is given below.

The FP10

NHS 'FP10' prescription forms were introduced in April 1998. For added security they are serially numbered and have anti-counterfeiting and anti-forgery features. Over the years there has been an increase in the number of different types of FP10 prescriptions. The main driver for this has been the expanding number of prescribing professionals.

Once FP10 prescriptions are printed they are purchased by Primary Care Trusts and hospitals and distributed free of charge to GPs, nurses, NHS dentists and other prescribers. To view the different types of FP10 see Table 6.2.

The situation is slightly different in Scotland and Wales where FP10GB and FP10HP prescriptions are used respectively; the latter was replaced by the bilingual W10HP in December 2003.

Private prescriptions

These prescriptions do not have to be written on particular forms and thus can be written, or computer generated, on an appropriate piece of paper. However, to comply with good clinical practice, the same general rules in the writing of a prescription should apply as detailed below. Once written, doctors are entitled to charge a fee in all cases except when prescribing Schedule 1 drugs (see below), where no charge can be made. No charge can also be made at any time for NHS prescriptions.

Writing a prescription – the 'nuts and bolts'

We have considered the types of prescription that various members of the primary healthcare team can use. Now we can look at how to actually generate a prescription.

It is a prescriber's duty to ensure that the prescriptions they write are clear and unambiguous. This was exemplified by the following case.[4] A doctor wrote a prescription for Amoxil tablets (amoxicillin) for a patient. The pharmacist misread this and dispensed Daonil (glibenclamide) instead. The patient was not a diabetic and unfortunately suffered permanent brain damage as a result of taking the drug. The court indicated that a doctor owed a duty of care to a patient to write a prescription clearly and with sufficient legibility to allow for possible mistakes by a busy pharmacist. The court concluded that the word Amoxil on the prescription could have been read as Daonil. It found that the doctor had been in breach of his duty to write clearly and thus had been negligent. The court also concluded that the doctor's failure to write clearly had contributed to the negligence of the pharmacist, although the greater proportion of the responsibility lay with the pharmacist. The implications of this ruling are that prescribers are under a legal duty of care to write clearly, with sufficient legibility to allow for mistakes by others. When illegible handwriting results in a breach of that duty, causing personal injury, then the courts will be prepared to punish the careless by awarding the appropriate damages.

A prescription must be dated, state the full name and address of the patient, and be signed by the prescriber. It is a legal duty to state the age of children under 12 years, but it is generally considered good practice to include the age and date of birth on all prescriptions. All writing should ideally be in ink and hence indelible. However, carbon copies are permissible as long as they are signed in ink.

Table 6.2: Different types of FP10 forms

Type	Use	Colour	Format
FP10C	Computer prescription – prescription and prescriber details printed by computer prescribing system	Green	Tractor feed printer forms. Box of 2000 forms
FP10NC	Handwritten prescription – prescriber details printed by manufacturer	Green	Pad of 50 forms
FP10SS	Computer single-sheet prescription – prescription and prescriber details printed by computer prescribing system	Green	Single-sheet printer forms. Box of 2000 forms Also used by other services, e.g. deputising
FP10MDA	GP Drug Misuse instalment prescription – prescriber details printed by manufacturer	Blue	Pad of 10 forms. A4 width not length. Handwritten controlled drug instalment prescriptions
FP10MDA-SS	Single-sheet Drug Misuse instalment prescription – prescription and prescriber details printed by computer prescribing system	Blue	Box of 500 forms. A4 width not length. For computer-produced drug instalment prescriptions. Only for doctors with handwriting exemption from Home Office
FP10P	Handwritten prescription pad. Prescriber details and type of prescriber, e.g. 'extended formulary nurse' printed by manufacturer	Lilac	Pad of 50 forms, supplied to nurse prescribers
FP10D	Community dentist prescriptions	Yellow	Pad of 50 forms
FP10HP	Hospital outpatient prescriptions	Peach	Top-stapled pads of 50 forms

To avoid dispensing confusion there are some particular areas that are worth mentioning.

1. The drug name should not be abbreviated. The generic name should not be used for modified-release medications and other special conditions due to the potential variation in plasma levels that could occur when varying products are dispensed.
2. Wherever possible decimal points should be avoided, e.g. instead of writing 0.1 gram, it is better practice to write 100 milligrams.
3. With even smaller amounts, such as micrograms, these should *not* be abbreviated.
4. The drug dose and frequency must be stated, or if the medication is 'As required', then the minimum dose interval should be stated. In the case of oral liquid preparations, volumes smaller than 5ml will be given by means of an oral syringe.
5. Dose directions should preferably be in English, though Latin abbreviations are used (see Table 6.3).
6. The quantity to be dispensed must be stated or the number of days of treatment inserted in the relevant box on the prescription.
7. The name of the medicine will appear on the label unless the prescriber indicates otherwise. If a prescriber does not wish a pharmacist to write the drug name on the label of the dispensed medication they can indicate this by writing the symbol 'NP' (*nomen proprium*, Latin for 'proper name') with a line through it (NP) on the prescription form. This gives the prescriber a choice of writing a description of the medication, e.g. 'sleeping tablets' instead of temazepam. The pharmacist will now not print the preparation name on that particular label. If a number of prescriptions are on one form, the prescriber can stipulate which is to be labelled with the drug name by writing the NP symbol only next to the items *not* to be labelled with the drug name. This can be useful for patients (or carers) who may not associate a drug name with its intended use.

Table 6.3: Latin abbreviations

Latin abbreviation	Latin	English
a.c.	Ante cibum	Before food
b.d.	Bis die	Twice daily
o.d.	Omni die	Once daily
o.m.	Omni mane	In the morning
o.n.	Omni nocte	At night
p.c.	Post cibum	After food
p.r.n.	Pro re nata	When required
q.d.s.	Quater die sumendus	Four times daily
q.q.h.	Quarta quaque hora	Every four hours
stat.	Stat	Immediately
t.d.s.	Ter die sumendus	Three times daily

Prescription endorsements

Schedule 2 is usually referred to as the Selected List. If one of these drugs is prescribed, the GP must endorse the face of the FP10 with the reference 'SLS' (Selected List Scheme). Another example of where a prescription endorsement is needed is in the prescribing of borderline substances. In this situation the prescription should be endorsed ACBS (Advisory Committee on Borderline Substances). It should be noted that endorsement by the prescriber in this instance is not absolutely necessary for the prescription to be supplied. However, this could be considered good practice as it shows that the prescriber has considered the above. Prescriptions issued in accordance with the Committee's advice and endorsed ACBS will normally not be investigated (see the Prescription Pricing Authority, Chapter 7).

Finally, if a woman requires a prescription for a contraceptive not on the List of Contraceptive Drugs to Be Dispensed Free of Charge (Part XVI – Notes on Charges, Drug Tariff), the prescription will have to be endorsed with a female symbol or 'for contraceptive use'. The prescription endorsements indicate to the Prescription Pricing Authority (see Chapter 7) that the dispensed item can be reimbursed under GMS Pharmaceutical Services.

There are instances where a pharmacist may endorse a prescription. An example may be where there is a prescription query where the pharmacist contacts the prescriber for clarification. If contact is made then the prescription is endorsed p.c. (prescriber contacted) by the pharmacist. If contact with the prescriber has not been possible and the pharmacist feels that it is appropriate to dispense a medication, then the prescription is endorsed p.n.c. (prescriber not contacted). Further exploration of pharmacist endorsements is outside the realms of this chapter. However, interested readers are directed towards the relevant reference.[5]

Computer-generated prescriptions

Over the last decade there has been a huge increase in the number of prescriptions that are computer generated. The general guidance offered by the General Practitioners Committee (of the British Medical Association) and the Royal College of General Practitioners has been accepted and implemented by the various software companies. This guidance, not surprisingly, is very similar to that described above for handwritten prescriptions. However, there are some differences that are worth considering.

The computer must print out the following: the patient's (not compulsory – see BNF) surname, one forename, other initials, address and the date. With regard to age, children under the age of 12 years and adults over the age of 60 years must have this printed in the appropriate box. Children under five years of age need their age printed in years and months. Printed at the bottom of the computer prescription form is the name of the responsible doctor, the surgery address, reference number, Health Authority and surgery telephone number.

The prescription must be printed in English without abbreviations, with the dose in numbers, the frequency in words and quantity in numbers, in brackets. In an attempt to reduce forgery the computer may print the number of prescriptions on the form. Handwritten alterations are to be discouraged and should be only carried out in rare circumstances. When this is required, the alteration has to be made by the prescriber and countersigned. Electronic signatures or stamps are not currently permitted on paper prescriptions. To allow the pilots for electronic transmission of prescriptions to go ahead in England, the Prescription Only Medicines Order has been amended to allow authorised prescribers who are participating in the pilot schemes to sign prescriptions digitally in place of ink signatures.

Great care must be taken by prescribers when using computers to generate prescriptions. The computer entry should not be abbreviated because inadvertent errors can easily occur. This occurred in a case where a doctor entered the abbreviation 'Penicil' into the computer, with the dose 250mg, frequency q.d.s. and quantity of 28 tablets. The issued and unfortunately dispensed drug was in fact penicillamine and not penicillin as intended.

Controlled drugs (CD)

These drugs are governed by the Misuse of Drugs Regulations 2001 and are specified in Schedules 2 (e.g. diamorphine, morphine and methadone) and 3 (temazepam and buprenorphine) of the NHS GMS Regulations. Controlled Drugs Schedules 4 (benzodiazepines and anabolic steroids) and 5 (codeine) also exist. The spotlight has been placed on this area of prescribing after the horrific case of mass murder carried out by Harold Shipman. The safeguards in place in the current system failed when it came to Shipman. He was able to obtain large quantities of CDs for his own purposes. Some of the patients he obtained diamorphine for were dead, some had no need for the drug and to others he gave only part of their supply that he had collected from the pharmacy. After a patient's death, he would collect any remaining supplies of CDs from their home and retain them for his own purposes. Certainly there are lessons to be learnt from this case and changes will follow on from the Shipman Inquiry. Readers are advised to update their prescribing knowledge once these changes are in place. However, detailed below are the present legal requirements for writing a prescription for a CD.

Prescriptions ordering CDs originally had to be in the prescriber's own handwriting in indelible ink and state:

1. The patient's name and address.
2. The strength and form of the preparation.
3. The total quantity of the preparation, or, if appropriate, the total number of units, in both words and figures. The only exception to this is prescriptions for temazepam.
4. The dose and modality of delivery, e.g. oral or subcutaneous.
5. For dentists the words 'For dental treatment only'.
6. The prescriber's signature and date.

Computer-generated prescriptions for CDs are now permissible. Points 1 to 5 above are in print whilst the signature and date have to be written by hand in indelible ink by the prescriber.

Prescriptions for CDs can be dispensed in instalments. When this is required the form FP10MDA (GP10 in Scotland) is used. The amount and intervals for the instalments must be specified for a period of up to 14 days. The prescription itself is only valid for 13 weeks from the date stated on the prescription, unlike a normal FP10 that is valid for up to six months. For a further consideration of the medicolegal aspects of controlled drugs see Chapter 10. Readers wanting a more in-depth consideration of controlled drug prescribing should reference the following website: www.dh.gov.uk/ PolicyAndGuidance/MedicinesPharmacyAndIndustry/Prescriptions/ControlledDrugs/ ControlledDrugsArticle/fs/en?CONTENT_ID=4131326&chk=dEgR/w.

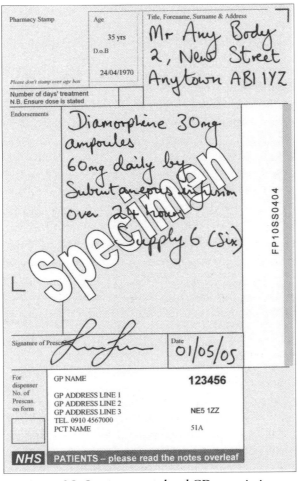

Figure 6.2: Specimen completed CD prescription

Drugs likely to cause dependence or misuse

Doctors have long had concerns with patients requesting drugs that can cause dependence or be misused. There have been many publications warning practitioners about the potential pitfalls in this area and hence this section would certainly not be complete without some consideration of this.

A prescriber has three main areas of responsibility:

- To avoid creating dependence by introducing drugs to patients without sufficient reason. It is known that a very large number of patients in the UK take tablets that neither do them much good nor much harm, but are committed to them indefinitely because they cannot easily be stopped.
- To ensure that the patient does not gradually increase the dose of a drug to the point where dependence becomes more likely. This tendency is seen especially with hypnotics and anxiolytics. A minimal amount should be prescribed in the first instance, or when seeing a new patient for the first time.
- To avoid being used as an unwitting source of supply for addicts. Methods include visiting more than one doctor, fabricating stories and forging prescriptions.

Responsibility

The responsibility for a prescription rests with the person who has written the script. This is irrespective of whether the patient is in a shared-care programme or not. Further considerations of the legal aspects of prescribing are made in Chapter 10. Another often-overlooked area of responsibility is in the security of prescribers' prescriptions. The most salient points for GPs to consider are as follows:

- Prescription forms are not to be left unattended at reception desks
- They are not to be left in a car where they may be visible
- When not in use, they should be kept in a locked drawer, whether this is at home or the place of work.

The lost prescription pad

To minimise the level of potential losses or thefts, prescribers are asked to keep only a small number of prescriptions in their possession. When thefts or losses do occur, prescribers should carry out the following tasks immediately on the discovery of that loss:

1. Inform the police
2. Inform the Primary Care Trust.

The Primary Care Trust will then initiate the notification of pharmacists and other general practitioners. It will also inform the Prescription Pricing Authority Fraud Investigation Unit. The relevant prescriber is advised to sign prescriptions in red for the following two months.

In this chapter we have looked at how to write a prescription. However, we must not lose sight of the fact that the central issue when writing a prescription is the patient. Careful attention to the generation of a prescription will reduce the potential for prescribing errors, the need for pharmacist queries and indeed dispensing errors. All these factors can improve the patient experience, at what is often a difficult time for ill patients.

References

1. Department of Health Statistics.
   www.dh.gov.uk/PublicationsAndStatistics/Publications/PublicationsPolicyAndGui
   dance/PublicationsPolicyAndGuidanceArticle/fs/en?CONTENT_ID=4088644&
   chk=FmBwZr [accessed May 2006].
2. *British National Formulary*. www.bnf.org/bnf/ [accessed May 2006].
3. National Health Service (General Medical Services Contracts) Regulations 2004.
   www.legislation.hmso.gov.uk/si/si2004/20040291.htm [accessed May 2006].
4. Aronson JK. Medication errors resulting from the confusion of drug names.
   Expert Opinion on Drug Safety May 2004; **3(3)**: 167–72.
5. The Prescription Pricing Authority. www.ppa.org.uk/edt/May_2005/mindex.htm
   [accessed May 2006].

The prescription pathway

Brian Crichton

This chapter charts the voyage of a prescription form as it leaves the doctor's consulting room, is endorsed by a dispensing pharmacist and is eventually processed by the Prescription Pricing Authority (PPA). This text allows a reader to gain an understanding of the various players and processes that are involved in this truly multifaceted journey.

Dispensing doctors

In the vast majority of practices in the UK, once a prescription has been written it is given to the patient. The patient can then choose which pharmacy to attend to get this dispensed. This, however, cannot occur in rural communities, as the nearest pharmacy may be many miles away. This would severely disadvantage patients, thus a doctors' practice in these instances not only generates the prescription but also dispenses the required medicines. Hence the term 'a dispensing practice' has been coined. The regulations around offering this service are that patients must live one or more miles away from a commercial dispensing pharmacy. This is not as the crow flies but by the distance travelled by road.[1] The only exception to this is for temporary residents.

Dispensing practices can only achieve this level of service with significant infrastructure in place. These practices will generally have a computer system, which can either print the prescription in the consulting room or send it electronically to the dispensary. This will of course depend on the patient's wishes, as they have a right to choose where to have their prescriptions dispensed. The majority, naturally enough, will choose the practice. At the dispensary most computer systems will print the prescription, print the medicine label and re-order the dispensed item, all in one go! This allows for much more efficient stock control. This process requires resources, which is offset by increased income from the rural practice allowance and the profit made from dispensing medicines. With regard to the latter, there is ongoing debate about whether there should be a move away from the 'on cost system' (profit made from the dispensed item), which provides an incentive for dispensing practices to prescribe expensive medications. This incentive occurs as, generally, bigger profits can be made from the more expensive items, which potentially creates an ethical dilemma. Consideration could be given to replacing this 'on cost system' with either a dispensing grant or a grant related to the number of items dispensed. This would address one of the major criticisms of dispensing.

Within dispensing practices there is currently considerable concern, since the funding is not seen as secure in the long term. This is fuelled by the example of Northern Ireland, where dispensing has been phased out throughout the province. However, it is clear that dispensing practices offer a tremendous added service for rural patients.

'Non-dispensing' practices do in fact dispense! They do this, however, on a much smaller scale. An example of this would be the bulk purchasing of influenza vaccine for the annual flu vaccination campaign. Large practices may be able to attract considerable discounts on bulk purchases and hence be able to achieve a profit, as they will be reimbursed by the PPA at the Drug Tariff price (profit = tariff price – purchase price).

The pharmacist

Once a prescription has been issued, whether it is by a dispensing or non-dispensing prescriber, the actual prescription is taken to a dispensing pharmacy. Once accepted the prescription goes through three phases:

1. *Professional assessment*. This is where the prescription is checked for the legality of the script, correct endorsements, any omissions, any mistakes, etc. This until recently was carried out exclusively by pharmacists. However, this can now be done by checking technicians who are to be qualified to National Vocational Qualification (NVQ) level 4.

2. *Dispensing*. This is the process by which the prescription request is translated into the required medication. This may simply require the retrieval off a shelf for a specified medication with the required number being dispensed. However, the process may be more complicated as is the case of mixing creams etc. Dispensing can be carried out by any one of the following, a pharmacist, a checking technician, a pharmacist dispensing technician (NVQ level 3) or a dispensing assistant (NVQ level 2). The exact complement of staff will generally be dependent on the volume of prescriptions passing through a pharmacy. The greater the volume the greater amount of staff needed.

3. *The final accuracy check*. This again can either be done by the pharmacist or checking technician. Ideally (though not a legal obligation) the final check should *not* be done by the person who did the dispensing. This reduces potential dispensing errors.

The training that has been put in place in pharmacies was catalysed by an unfortunate incident involving a prescription for peppermint water. The details of this tragic case are as follows. 'The Alder Hey peppermint water case'[2] involved a baby named Matthew Young, a resident in Runcorn, Cheshire, who in 1998 was inadvertently dispensed peppermint water that was made up with concentrated chloroform water instead of double-strength chloroform water, resulting in the death of the baby from cardiorespiratory arrest due to chloroform inhalation. The ripples of this case were felt across the whole of the pharmacy profession, where important lessons were learnt.

Once medicines are dispensed they are then passed back again to the pharmacist for final checking prior to being given to the patient. The training required in order to be a pharmacist has been considered in Chapter 4.

It is worth at this point pausing to consider the various charges that occur both for the NHS and patients. This will enable us to understand how pharmacists are remunerated and which patients are indeed exempt from prescription charges.

The dispensing of a prescription attracts the following fees:

- Professional fee.
- Container allowance. For the container, or spoon/syringe for liquids etc.
- Drug or appliance cost.
- Special fees. For example the measuring of a patient for surgical stockings.
- Additional fees. An example would be mixing of ingredients, e.g. 2 per cent menthol in aqueous cream. The calculations, weights and details of the mixtures have to be entered into a book called 'The extemporaneous dispensing and special procurements book'. This has to be signed by the dispenser and pharmacist, i.e. double-checked.

There is a 'claw-back scheme', which attempts to reduce the effect of increased profits, as higher-turnover pharmacies are able to obtain larger discounts from wholesalers. Thus the larger the turnover the greater the 'claw-back'.

New sets of fees are being negotiated for pharmacists undertaking new duties, e.g. patients' blood pressure measurement, electronic prescribing (see Chapter 9), etc. However, readers requiring a more detailed understanding are directed towards the Drug Tariff.

For private prescriptions the situation is different. The pharmacist receiving the private prescription will charge the patient a sum made up of these various components:

- dispensing fee
- special or additional fees
- drug cost plus 'mark-up'.

The total cost may vary as a patient moves from one pharmacy to another, as there are no statutes governing the charging structure. Some pharmacies have a minimum charge, e.g. £4 might be levied even if the drug cost was merely a few pence. The pharmacist for audit purposes keeps the private prescription and it thus travels no further.

The Drug Tariff

The Drug Tariff is a volume that is produced monthly by the Pharmaceutical Directorate of the PPA for the Secretary of State and is supplied primarily to pharmacists, doctors' surgeries and (twice yearly) nurse prescribers. The text is produced as a hard copy or via the internet.[3] It tells individuals the rules that should be followed when dispensing, the value of the fees and allowances paid, and what's allowed. One has to remember that the Drug Tariff does not account for all drugs, e.g. modified-release medicines, but lists the drugs included according to the appropriate *British National Formulary* (BNF) chapter. The costs of the drugs held within this volume are calculated by the DoH by looking at the drug costs across a range of major wholesalers and then taking an average. This constitutes the 'Drug Tariff price'.

Prescription exemption

Some 85 per cent of all the prescriptions dispensed in 1999 were exempt from the standard prescription charge. In fact the prescription charge exemption arrangements are still among the most liberal in Europe. Below is a list of patients who are eligible for prescription exemption:

- under 16 years of age
- under 19 years of age and in full-time education
- 60 years of age or older
- holds a current maternity exemption certificate (FP92)
- holds a current medical exemption certificate (FP92A)
- holds a current prescription pre-payment certificate (FP96)
- has a war pension exemption certificate
- named on the current HC2 charges certificate
- prescribed free-of-charge contraceptive
- obtains income support
- obtains jobseeker's allowance
- holds a working families' tax credit NHS exemption certificate
- holds a disabled person's tax credit NHS exemption certificate.

From the medical point of view we can consider those illnesses that qualify for prescription exemption. Generally they are those that require some form of replacement therapy, but not exclusively. Listed below are the medical conditions eligible for prescription exemption:

- epilepsy
- diabetes mellitus requiring drug therapy
- hypothyroidism
- hypoparathyroidism
- diabetes insipidus or other forms of hypopituitarism

- myasthenia gravis
- hypoadrenalism requiring replacement therapy, e.g. Addison's disease
- permanent fistula requiring dressings or appliances
- a 'continuing physical disability' with the inability to go out (i.e. travel outside of the home) without the help of another person.

One can certainly debate the criteria for exemption. However, further to this, one could argue over whether an individual with an exempted condition should have exemption to all prescription charges, rather than just prescriptions pertaining to that particular condition. A full exploration of this issue is outside the boundaries of this book.

Prescription pre-payment

It is possible for patients to pay a single fee 'up-front' to enable prescription charge exemption for a variable time period. A prescription pre-payment certificate (FP96) is issued in these instances and can be obtained from a dispensing pharmacy or online from the PPA.[4] This becomes worthwhile for our patients if they require more than five prescriptions in a four-month period, or more than 14 prescriptions in a 12-month period.

Pharmacists are obliged to ask for evidence of exemption from prescription charges. However, the medicines can still be dispensed without this evidence. In these cases there is a box on the back of the prescription saying 'Evidence not seen'. A cross placed in this box will trigger targeting by the PPA Fraud Investigation Unit (see below). Thus the pharmacist is in no way responsible for the accuracy of the patient's declaration; this remains the patient or carer's responsibility.

Urgent dispensing

Urgent dispensing occurs when a patient has a prescription that needs to be dispensed during 'unsociable hours'. This rare event is becoming even rarer as we see the growth in 24-hour centres and most doctors carry a small supply of emergency medications to cover these types of situations. However, if a patient urgently requires a medication, which is not available by other means, then there is a duty pharmacist within each designated area that can be called upon in these instances.

Once medications are dispensed, pharmacists have to collect all the prescriptions together and send them to the relevant PPA office to be processed.

The PPA

The PPA occupies an important position within the NHS. The work carried out by this department is fundamental to the payment for drugs dispensed and budget setting by many professionals involved in direct patient care. The throughput is huge, with a staggering 608 million prescription items processed in 2001/02. The full scope of the PPA can only be appreciated by considering its main functions. These lie in four main areas:

- to calculate and make payments for drugs and appliances provided under the NHS
- to provide prescribing information for primary care in terms of volume, costs and trends
- to manage a range of health benefits, e.g. maternity benefits etc.
- to produce the Drug Tariff.

Prescriptions received by the PPA are processed so that the correct pharmacists and dispensing doctors are paid what is due. The prescribing number on each prescription is read so that the cost of each item can be set against the drug budget for an individual practice and prescriber. The prescribing information is published in many forms, but of particular interest to primary care is the quarterly published Prescribing Analysis and Cost (PACT) data report. For more information with regard to PACT data, readers are directed towards Chapter 9.

A diagrammatic representation of the prescription pathway is shown in Figure 7.1.

Tackling fraud

The NHS constitutes a massive employer with a huge turnover. Unfortunately, as a result of this it is open to fraud. Individual cases in the lay or specialised medical press where fraud and theft have been uncovered abound, sometimes involving very substantial sums of money. To help combat these cases the NHS has created the NHS Counter Fraud Service (DCFS).

By the end of August 2002 the DCFS was investigating 414 cases of suspected fraud involving 470 individuals and potentially £18.8 million! Looking more closely at these cases showed they included 82 GPs, 18 hospital doctors, 44 dentists, 43 opticians, 101 pharmacists, 106 NHS employees, 29 external contractors or suppliers, and 18 patients. This highlights the extent of opportunity for fraud that lies within the NHS.

The most serious cases that have been examined to date include:

- an optician who claimed more than £750,000 for sight tests on non-existent or dead people
- a dentist who is alleged to have claimed more than £2 million for work that had simply not been done
- a dispensing GP who claimed more that £1 million for drugs, which were not actually dispensed
- several multi-million pound frauds by external contractors.

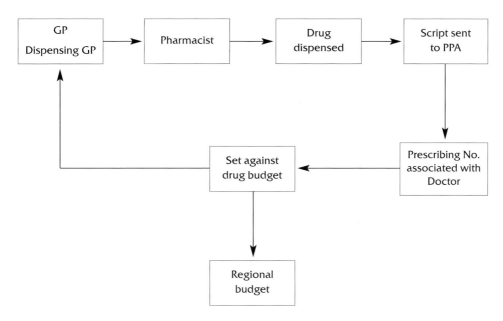

Figure 7.1: The prescription pathway

The DCFS

The DCFS was originally set up in September 1998 with a remit to counter all fraud and corruption in the NHS with a specific priority for countering fraud in the Family Health Services. It actually started to function in April 1999 and has already cut losses from patient prescription fraud by £48 million! Dental checks started in November 2000 and have cut losses due to dental patient fraud by 25 per cent, i.e. £30 million.

The DCFS checks for opticians came into force in February 2001. Now when a patient claims they are entitled to NHS sight tests or vouchers they are asked for proof that they do not indeed have to pay. Cases are being investigated and anyone found to have claimed incorrectly will face a penalty charge of up to £100, and, in some cases, prosecution.

A confidential telephone hotline was set up in December 2000 that allows NHS staff and patients to report any suspicion of fraud or corruption. The NHS fraud and corruption reporting line can be contacted on 08702 400100.

The introduction of a proof of exemption clause on the standard prescription form – checked by pharmacists before people receive their medicines – has paid immediate dividends. Losses to patient prescription charge fraud were reduced from £117 million in 1998 to £69 million the following year, i.e. a reduction of £48 million. To date 126 successful criminal prosecutions have been undertaken along with more than 184 successful civil and disciplinary cases.

In this chapter we have tracked the passage of a prescription as it moves along 'the prescription pathway'. It is clear that many professionals are involved in this process with the role of the PPA in quality control and 'horizon planning', which are of vital importance. When one looks to the future to make plans for expenditure on prescribing, whether at a national, Primary Care Trust (PCT) or practice level, one needs to understand some of the basic principles of economics. It is to this that we now turn in the next chapter.

References

1. National Health Service (General Medical Services Contracts) Regulations 2004. www.legislation.hmso.gov.uk/si/si2004/20040291.htm [accessed May 2006].
2. Editorial. Peppermint water case settlement. *Pharmaceutical Journal* 3 June 2000; **264(7099)**: 832.
3. The Drug Tariff. www.ppa.org.uk/edt/May_2005/mindex.htm [accessed May 2006].
4. The Prescription Pricing Authority. www.ppa.org.uk/index.htm [accessed May 2006].

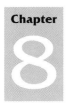

Chapter 8

Health economics and prescribing

Tom Walley

Money and medicines

Health services throughout the world are increasingly faced with new demands for health care. However, as this demand grows, so too do the resource constraints faced by decision makers. In most European countries, the costs of prescribing are borne in large part by the state in one form or another. Since states get their funding from taxation and no one likes to pay taxes, the state has to spend the taxpayers' money in a responsible way and be able to demonstrate this. The costs of prescribing in particular rise year on year, ahead of the rate of general inflation, ahead of the rate of tax increases, and ahead of the high rates of even medical inflation. Examples of the rates of rise are shown in Figure 8.1.

Small wonder then that states try to contain the rise in prescribing costs in a variety of ways, or that they try to ensure that the best health gain is achieved for every pound or euro spent. No country really expects that they can actually reduce the costs of prescribing.

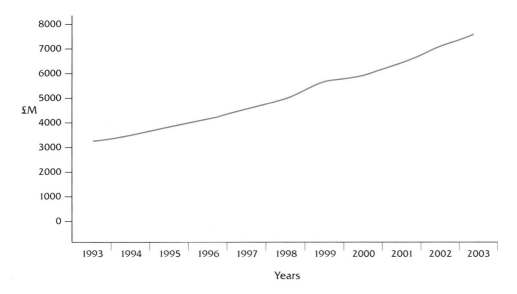

Figure 8.1: The rising drug bill in primary care (England, 1993–2003)

This chapter therefore examines several issues in relation to money and prescribing, under two broad headings. The first is the 'accountancy' or budgets related to prescribing: how much does it cost, and where does the money go; and how is it managed. GPs may recognise this as prescribing budgeting. The second is health economics and how that is assessed and applied in relation to prescribing. These two are related but not the same; the difference between the two is that accountancy allows for expenditures and managing the expenditures, but doesn't consider the benefits achieved by prescribing. It also involves real money! Health economics tries to consider both costs (in the widest sense) and benefits, and is inevitably more theoretical. I will try to draw these two strands together at the end. Although these problems are common all over the world, this chapter will consider only the UK NHS.

Budgets and prescribing

Money for prescribing in primary care in the UK comes from the unified or single budget given to primary care organisations (PCOs). There is no independent budget line for prescribing, although for accounting purposes PCOs may talk about a prescribing 'budget' – this is just a notional budget set aside on paper for prescribing costs in a given year but any money spent on prescribing takes money away from other services, and any money saved can be put back into other services.

Community prescribing typically accounts for 14 per cent of a PCO's total budget,[1] around £151 per head in England in 2003, and more in Scotland and Wales. But prescribing differs from other areas in that the NHS effectively guarantees all spending on prescribing – when a doctor writes a prescription, the NHS guarantees that it will pay the cost of that prescription to the dispensing pharmacist, regardless of where the money comes from. This kind of open-ended guarantee does not exist for any other area of healthcare spending. It may also undermine other areas of health care; for instance, a PCO may plan to spend money on a new service, but it cannot really control spending on prescribing. This is why PCOs put so much effort into prescribing issues. Of course, they recognise the great benefits that prescribing effective medicines to the right patients may bring, and that often this is a highly efficient use of healthcare resources.

Hospital prescribing comes out of the overall hospital budget, largely in turn from the PCO unified budget. So, in the past, hospitals tried to save money on their budget by making special deals to buy drugs very cheaply from companies who would recoup their profits by higher prices in the community, or 'dumped' prescribing of high-cost drugs onto the GP (and out of the hospital budget). Now PCOs exert pressure on hospitals to consider the community costs of prescribing, e.g. in their choice of drug, since any great overspend on prescribing may undermine hospital as well as primary care services.

If a PCO does exceed its expected spending on medicines, its options are to take money from other services or to set it against next year's budget – in effect taking a mortgage against next year's money that will have to be repaid at some point.

A key issue for the PCO is how its overall budget is set. This is done partly on the basis of historical spending and partly on a complex equation that takes into account the number of patients, their age (the old and the very young require more medical services), mortality rates (used because we don't have good data on rates of illness) and poverty. This budget setting is controversial since changes in the formula used may advantage or disadvantage many areas. However, from 2001 onwards, NHS prescribing budgets have been growing at a rate of 10–11 per cent per year and some of the major pressures now come from attempts to implement government directives such as the National Institute for Health and Clinical Excellence (NICE) guidance or National Service Frameworks.

The PCO may issue practices with notional practice budgets for prescribing. These are only paper budgets, and are used only for monitoring and for comparing practices. These budgets are set in different PCOs in a variety of ways – there is a national formula, which puts most weight on numbers of patients with an age and morbidity allowance. However, many PCOs choose to use a combination of this and of historical spending, arguing that budgets would be unrealistic and ignored if they expect changes that are too drastic.

Once the practice 'budget' is set, spending in each year is monitored against this and the GPs will receive monthly reports of their expenditure against this budget from the Prescription Pricing Authority (in England). There are no penalties for overspending against this budget, but PCOs have operated inventive schemes, and some encourage GPs to contain their spending within the budget. These are now mostly wrapped up in overall quality payments.

A key problem in setting budgets at a practice level is that the formulae used are derived from averages, and individual practice may differ, dependent on their particular mix of patients in terms of age and illness. This means that budgets might be inadequate for some practices, but too generous for others. The counter to this is that since these budgets are only indicative or theoretical, this doesn't matter.

From the PCO point of view, they too are at risk in their planning because they don't really know what prescribing is going to be in the next year, though they will try hard to predict. It could be particularly affected by a new drug coming on the market, or NICE advice about an expensive drug, which it has to fund.

So how will PCOs try to manage their prescribing budgets? First of all they have to make sure that enough money comes in – by making a sufficiently strong case for funding overall, and, within the PCO, the prescribing team have to argue for an appropriate notional allocation to prescribing.

Then they must try to control expenditures wherever reasonable, i.e. without causing harm to patient care. A simple example of this is generic prescribing; where a generic drug is available it is usually much less expensive than the market leader. The Drug Tariff sets the NHS price for most generics; this is based on the list prices of generics, but is often slow to change. In general, companies are allowed to set their own prices for branded products but the government controls the price of key generics. Some branded generic preparations may in the short term be less expensive than the Drug Tariff price, and some advocate their use for this reason. However, this requires that the prescriber keeps a close eye on changing prices of the branded preparations and the Drug Tariff. Most regard this as too much trouble for the return, and it undermines the clinical virtues of generic prescribing, which are clear.

PCOs will also suggest therapeutic substitutions of drugs, e.g. changing a more expensive drug in a class for a cheaper alternative. An example of this is replacing atorvastatin with simvastatin, which is fine for most (but perhaps not all) patients. It is always up to the prescriber to decide whether such substitutions are reasonable, but it is also the prescriber's responsibility to avoid any unnecessary waste of NHS resources.[2] PCOs will therefore try to help doctors to have some awareness of the costs of their prescribing.

PCOs will also try to counter the influence of the pharmaceutical industry by promoting access to and use of unbiased information about therapeutics.

What PCOs and GPs cannot often do, except in a superficial way, is to take a wider view of what is truly cost-effective in prescribing, i.e. where a new drug increases benefits but also increase costs, the question is whether that is good value for money. This is the role of health economics, and the skills to do this are in short supply. For the NHS in England, this function is centralised in NICE. Scotland and Wales have parallel systems.

Before we look at the role of NICE, therefore, we need to understand a little about how the cost-effectiveness of a medicine is evaluated.

Health economics and prescribing

Every health service in the world lacks enough resources to do everything that is possible. Choices have to be made therefore about allocation of resources. Health economics seeks to inform these choices, by weighing the benefits of a healthcare intervention against its cost, not to save money, but to make the use of resources and the consequences of alternative use of these resources absolutely clear. In this way health economics can encourage more efficient use of limited healthcare resources. Pharmacoeconomics is no more than the application of health economics to medicines.

Health economics is about making choices between options, and is fundamentally *comparative*. So when we hear that 'drug x is cost effective', our immediate response should be 'compared with what?' Health economics is sometimes misused to support marketing ploys, and one way to bias the results of a study is to pick an unfavourable comparator. There is debate about what the ideal comparator should be – should it be the drug and dose most widely used for a condition, or a 'gold standard' comparator as defined in clinical trials? This raises further questions about the sources of medical evidence used in economic studies. Where possible, the studies should be based on strong medical evidence, but more importantly on what would actually happen in real-life medical practice, rather than in a clinical trial. But there is often little evidence available about the latter, and we are forced to make *assumptions* to fill the gaps due to our lack of knowledge. These assumptions should be reasonable, and should be quite clear, so that they can be challenged. Indeed any good economic study will challenge these assumptions itself, by varying them in a *sensitivity analysis*.

A sensitivity analysis explores the extent to which a conclusion is dependent on factors that have been assumed or about which there is controversy, e.g. clinical benefits. For instance, if a study uses a rate of relapse of duodenal ulcers after treatment of 5 per cent at one year, based on a clinical trial, it may make an assumption that the rate in real life will be the same. But what happens if in real life the relapse rate is actually 10 per cent or 1 per cent? These might drastically affect the outcome of a study. A sensitivity analysis is essential in any good economic evaluation to confirm to the reader that the results of the evaluation are robust, and to clarify what are the critical assumptions. It is important to remember that economic evaluations can only be as good as the clinical evidence they are based on; the weaker the clinical evidence, the more the health economist is forced into more assumptions (some assumptions are always inevitable), and the less reliable the results.

A number of other concepts are crucial in health economic evaluations and can be defined here:

Efficiency

This means deriving maximum benefit (i.e. health gain) from limited resources.

Opportunity cost

This is defined as the 'benefit forgone when selecting one therapy alternative over the next best alternative'. What is of concern to us is not how much a healthcare intervention costs, but what we are giving up to use that intervention. This is a concept familiar to all of us, though not perhaps under this title. For instance, suppose I can afford to either buy a new car or to take an expensive holiday. The opportunity cost of buying one is my inability to enjoy the benefits of the other. If we spend £8 billion a year on the drug bill, what else might we spend that money on? And would it bring greater benefit if we did spend that money differently?

Incremental analysis

There is usually a current treatment for most conditions, with associated costs and benefits. Economic evaluations should focus on the costs and the benefits of a new intervention *over and above* those of our current therapy. For instance, consider the management of hypertension. We already have treatments for this (e.g. thiazides), but perhaps they can be improved on by using newer medicines (angiotensin 2 receptor blockers). We would not be advocating abandoning all existing treatment for blood pressure, so the question is not what are the costs and benefits of the new drugs in hypertension, but what are the added costs and benefit of using the new drugs, over and above costs and benefits obtained from existing drugs. (Since the new drugs have not been shown to be more effective than the older drugs, and are a lot dearer, this is an easy one to work out.)

This gives rise to a second, related concept of *marginal costs*. For instance, if a new treatment enables patients to be discharged from hospital a day earlier than they would otherwise, it might be tempting to put the average cost of a hospital bed day as a saving of resources. But however this new treatment worked, all the fixed-capital charges for a hospital bed that go into the average cost, e.g. costs of laboratories, kitchens and building maintenance, will be largely unchanged. The only costs that change may be those of having a patient physically occupy the bed – the costs of the patient's meals, treatment and perhaps nursing time. These are the marginal costs, where the resource used actually changes substantially. Incremental analysis is concerned with the marginal and not the average costs. Marginal costs are often very difficult to measure, and there is a temptation to use average costs instead. This may be justified if, for instance, enough bed days are saved by the widespread adoption of a new treatment to actually reduce bed numbers and to close wards.

Methods of economic evaluation

The various types of economic evaluations have a common structure in that they involve explicit measurement of inputs ('costs') and outcomes ('benefits') around medical interventions. Some outcomes might actually be costs (e.g. adverse drug reactions). Economic evaluation is essentially a framework that draws up a balance sheet between costs and benefits to assist decision making (Figure 8.2).

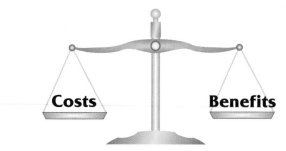

Figure 8.2: Health economics – balancing costs against benefits

Costs here mean not just the acquisition cost of a drug, or even all monetary costs, but may also include costs in the widest sense, including time lost from work, and distress. These costs might be:

- *Direct* – paid directly by the health service, including staff costs, capital costs and drug acquisition costs. We often use a reference set of NHS prices that are available as a short cut to look at these.
- *Indirect* – costs experienced by the patient (or family or friends) or society; for example, these might include loss of earnings, loss of productivity, loss of leisure time, cost of travel to hospital, etc. Many of these are difficult to measure, but should be of concern to society as a whole.
- *Intangible* – these are the pain, worry or other distress that a patient or their family might suffer. These may be impossible to measure in monetary terms, or even at all, and so are rarely considered in economic evaluations. Nevertheless, they are a concern for both doctors and patients.

The benefits we expect from an intervention might be measured in:

- *'Natural' units* – e.g. years of life saved, strokes prevented, ulcers healed, etc.
- *'Utility' units* – utility is an economist's word for satisfaction, or sense of wellbeing, and is an attempt to evaluate the quality of a state of health, and not just its quantity. Such utility measurements are therefore based on some measurement of quality of life, i.e. the physical, social and emotional aspects of the patient's wellbeing, which are not readily measured in physical terms. The methods of measurement of quality of life are controversial, but commonly used tools include the Short Form 36 questionnaire, or particularly popular at present the EuroQol (EQ-5) questionnaire. Some of these are unique to a single disease area, but some are more generic and can be used across a range of diseases.
- *The Quality Adjusted Life Year (QALY)* – one widely used utility measure. This is a relative summary of quality and quantity of life. It multiplies years of life by quality of life. For instance, if one's quality of life with angina is measured or judged to be 80 per cent of that a similar patient without angina, then a year of life for that angina patient would be 0.8 QALY. Imagine a treatment that could restore that patient to full quality of life (1 year = 1 QALY) at a cost of £20,000. The patient's life expectancy is four years. The health gain is 0.2 QALY × 4 = 0.8 QALY, and the cost per QALY gained would be £20,000/0.8 = £25,000. Suppose that as well as relieving the angina, the treatment also extended the patient's life expectancy to 6 years; now the health gain is (0.2 × 4) + (1 × 2) = 2.8 QALY, and the cost per QALY is £20,000/2.8 = £7142. This begs the question how much are we prepared to pay for a QALY worth, and we'll come back to this example when we talk about NICE.

Associated economic benefit – this is usually measured in money, which is a useful common denominator allowing comparisons across different disciplines. This measure includes, for instance, the economic benefits of returning someone to work.

Common types of study

These costs and benefits give rise to the four common types of economic evaluation.

Cost minimisation analysis (CMA)

This involves measuring only costs, usually only to the health service, and is applicable only where the health benefits are absolutely identical and therefore need not be considered separately, e.g. generic prescribing, or perhaps using enalapril or lisinopril to treat hypertension.

Cost-effectiveness analysis (CEA)

The term cost-effectiveness is often used loosely to refer to the whole of economic evaluation, but should strictly refer to one particular type of evaluation, in which the health benefit can be defined and measured in natural units (e.g. years of life saved, ulcers healed, fractures avoided), and the costs are measured in money. It therefore compares therapies with similar outcomes (although perhaps different success rates). For instance, if our desired outcome were reducing the risk of osteoporotic fracture in low-risk elderly patients, we could consider the costs per fracture avoided by using a bisphosphonate or by using vitamin D and calcium. CEA is the most commonly applied form of economic analysis in the literature, and especially in drug therapy. It does not allow comparisons to be made between two totally different areas of medicine, where there are different outcomes.

Cost utility analysis (CUA)

This is similar to cost-effectiveness in that there is a defined outcome and the cost to reach that outcome is measured in money. However, here the outcome is a unit of utility (e.g. a QALY).

Since the end point may not be directly dependent on the disease state, CUA can in theory look at more than one area of medicine, e.g. cost per QALY for coronary artery bypass grafting versus cost per QALY in using erythropoietin in pre-dialysis renal disease. In practice this is not so easy since the QALY is not a well-defined fixed unit transferable from study to study. Nevertheless, this is NICE's preferred way to evaluate drugs because it provides a similar base to look across all areas of medical intervention, and in theory allows it to compare the best use of resources in a whole range of areas.

Cost–benefit analysis (CBA)

Here, the benefit is measured as the associated economic benefit of an intervention, and hence both costs and benefits are expressed in money. CBA may ignore many intangible but very important benefits that are difficult to measure in monetary terms, e.g. relief of anxiety. CBA may also seem to discriminate against those in whom a return to productive employment is unlikely, e.g. the elderly, or the unemployed. For these reasons, this approach is not used much in health economics, although many purist economists like it on theoretical grounds and because it removes some of the 'sacred cow' protection that surrounds health care. They argue that health should be another commodity, and not necessarily valued more than other possible uses of the resources.

Further points

There are two further points that require definition.

Perspective

This asks from whose point of view is the study conducted – from that of the NHS where only direct costs are considered, or societal where indirect costs are studied as well. In general, the societal perspective is considered the more appropriate, but a healthcare manager with a limited budget might be tempted to ignore the societal view and consider only the costs that fall on their own budget. A study of migraine, which took the health service perspective, only might suggest that sumatriptan in migraine (a very high-cost drug in an area that previously cost the health service very little) was highly undesirable, but a study taking a societal perspective might come to the opposite conclusion. NICE usually adopts the perspective of the NHS and the publicly funded social services, but not a full societal perspective.

Discounting

There is often a difference in timing between the investment of health service resources and gaining the benefits. Therefore we must discount future spending etc. to try to equalise the effects of inflation and health and financial preferences over a long period. In general, costs are discounted at a rate set by the Treasury (currently 3.5 per cent). There is some debate over whether benefits should also be discounted. (It is relatively easy to accept that £100 spent now is worth more than £100 in five years' time, but how does one compare a healthy year now to a healthy year in five years' time?) NICE requires the discounting of both at present.

Limits of pharmacoeconomic evaluation

Many problems limit our ability to use health economics in the health service. The whole process may be viewed as open to bias. Bias may occur in the choice of comparator drug, the assumptions made where accurate data is lacking and in the selective reporting of results. The suspicion of bias arises because most studies are conducted or funded by pharmaceutical companies who obviously are interested in the results, and there is a publication bias towards those studies favourable to sponsoring companies. NICE tries to manage this by having its economic evaluations conducted by independent academic units.

Doctors may tend to equate health economics with rationing or cost-cutting, and fail to see that, for instance, health economics may expose under-funding (one of the reasons perhaps why NICE guidance has been generally so liberal in approving more spending in most areas it has looked at). Many doctors therefore reject on principle the whole process and refuse to consider it. While much of this does not stand up to serious thought, there is a potential conflict between the traditional Hippocratic medical ethic (my patient always deserves the best) and utilitarian ethics (what is best for this population of patients). The tensions in this are clear and are unlikely to be resolved, but can be constructive in advancing our thinking on the future of health services. The reality is that since resources are limited within the NHS, waste of resources by inefficiency is not ethical.[3] Inefficiency reduces clinicians' ability to give the best possible care to their patient. Far from being unethical to consider the economics of a medical intervention, it seems unethical not to.

NICE

NICE was set up for a number of reasons but there are two that concern us here: to promote equity in access to services across the NHS and to evaluate what interventions were cost-effective and should be introduced into the NHS (or sometimes in what circumstances the NHS should introduce a new technology, e.g. to which particular patients). The first problem of equity was seen in 'postcode prescribing' where different health authorities came to different decisions about access to some expensive services, because of their differing budgets, priorities and local assessments. This led to variations in what was available to patients and was politically unacceptable in a truly national service. When NICE guidance was first introduced many health authorities either continued to ignore it or delayed its adoption. From 2002, the secretary of state ordered that health authorities and later PCOs must make available the resources to deliver NICE guidance within three months of its issue. While this may seem to have resolved many of the equity problems, it created many more as we shall see below.

The second role of considering new technologies is based on an assessment of the clinical evidence to support its use, and a health economic evaluation, usually of the cost utility type. These are conducted for NICE independently. But the assessment may inevitably be weak in some areas – there may be relatively limited clinical evidence about a new therapy, and the health economics may involve some heroic extrapolations – e.g. if a drug treats a surrogate of disease, demonstrated in short-term trial (e.g. white cell count in chronic myeloid leukaemia in a trial of six weeks), what will that mean clinically and economically if the drug is given indefinitely? Furthermore, assessments based on health economics may not be enough – health services do not exist to be efficient: there are issues of fairness to patients, compassion where no other treatment is available (even if it is not cost-effective), practicality, etc. So NICE uses the assessment as part of its appraisal, but the appraisal will always involve value judgements. This is an example of health economics informing but not making decisions.

A key judgement is how much is a QALY worth? NICE rejects the idea of working to a formal threshold value, although in practice if an intervention costs less than £30,000 per QALY it will be accepted. If more than this, then it may not necessarily be rejected but its chances of acceptance diminish rapidly. Where did the figure of £30,000 come from? By looking at the cost/QALY of a range of things in the NHS that we all agree are worth doing, and therefore we implicitly accept this as a cost/QALY that we are willing to pay.

Even if something is cost effective but very expensive, there may not be enough money available in the system to pay for it. This is an issue of *affordability*, and NICE is not permitted to consider this. Affordability is a political decision, of how much money there is in the health service, and so the secretary of state reserves to himself or herself the decision about whether NICE recommendations should be accepted by the NHS and whether they are affordable. So far, the secretary of state has only limited the transfer of NICE advice to the NHS on one occasion – limiting the support for *in vitro* fertilisation.

To date, NICE has generally encouraged the uptake of new technologies and increased NHS costs; this may be acceptable when NHS budgets are growing, but budgets will not grow indefinitely and more difficult times may lie ahead. There is a danger that effective but unevaluated areas and services get pushed out as a result, and that more and more of the NHS budget gets sucked into new pharmaceuticals, simply because they have been evaluated when other services have not. The concept of NICE was feared initially by pharmaceutical companies, who saw it as a probable block to their market penetration; in practice, most companies are now keen to have a NICE guidance on their drug, being fairly confident that it will support its use rather than limit it.

Where theory and reality meet: the PCO budget

Now we can come back to where we started, and look at where the theory of the health economics considered by NICE, and the guidance based on that, meets the cold reality of NHS budgets. PCOs have to work within their constrained budgets while at the same time providing the resource to meet NICE guidance, and encouraging GPs to put this guidance into practice. The government has taken the view that the general increased funding to the NHS is enough to pay for the delivery of NICE guidance, and no further specific money is provided. In practice NICE guidance has been one of the biggest drivers of the rise in the drugs bill for some years, and seems set to continue. For the PCOs, this means that they have often to cut back or not develop other services, and that setting and delivering local priorities are often overtaken by NICE's priorities. There is therefore a balancing act for PCOs and for doctors to manage prescribing, so that the best health gain comes from money spent on it.

The results are usually even more pressure on the budgets. Many managers and professionals in the NHS have expressed disquiet that NICE has, as they see it, failed to control the tide of new medicines, many of uncertain value, and that NICE rates effectiveness perhaps over affordability and does not consider the consequences and opportunity costs of some of its decisions. This reduces confidence in NICE. This would be unfortunate since the role of NICE is clearly vital to the NHS.

Conclusions

Prescribing costs are rising and this rise has an opportunity cost, i.e. when we spend on medicines, we cannot spend the same money on something else. We recognise the great benefits that prescribing effective medicines to the right patients may bring and that often this is a highly efficient use of healthcare resources. To achieve this we must first ensure that there is as little waste as possible in our prescribing – it must cost as much as it needs to be effective but no more, and generic prescribing and careful drug selection are part of this. Second, we must ensure that, when we prescribe, money could not be better spent elsewhere; this is the role of health economic evaluation, and while we should all understand the basics of this, the techniques are beyond most of us. We must therefore look to a national body like NICE for their evaluations of this. However, these bodies need to give more concern to the affordability of their advice and its practicality. Third, we (both as individuals and corporately within a PCO) must always remember our responsibilities are to our patients. Squaring the many demands on us is never easy.

References
1. Worcestershire Primary Care drug budget. www.worcestershirehealth.nhs.uk [accessed May 2006].
2. National Health Service (General Medical Services Contracts) Regulations 2004. www.legislation.hmso.gov.uk/si/si2004/20040291.htm [accessed May 2006].
3. Excessive prescribing costs. Schedule 46. National Health Service (General Medical Services Contracts) Regulations 2004. www.legislation.hmso.gov.uk/si/si2004/20040291.htm [accessed May 2006].

Further reading
Walley T, Haycox A and Boland A (eds). *Pharmacoeconomics*. Edinburgh: Churchill Livingstone, 2004.

9 Monitoring prescribing

Brian Crichton and Fiona Beadle

Prescribers have a duty to ensure that the medicines they prescribe are safe, appropriate and cost-effective. The NHS spends over £8.6 billion each year on medicines and, of that, at least £100 million worth of medicines are returned to pharmacies for destruction.[1,2] Estimates of the number of hospital admissions due to problems with medicines range from 6 per cent to 10 per cent. This degree of waste and morbidity shows us clearly that monitoring prescribing is a very important part of medicines management in primary care.

Audit Commission report on primary care prescribing

According to the Audit Commission report,[3] in 2001/02 an average Primary Care Trust (PCT) spent £18 million on prescribing, representing about 16 per cent of its total expenditure. This is likely to rise, especially in areas covered by National Service Frameworks (NSFs), guidance issued by the National Institute for Health and Clinical Excellence (NICE) and the new 2004 General Medical Services (GMS) Contract. Information from the Prescribing Support Unit shows that the NSF for coronary heart disease is the most significant factor driving the increase in drug expenditure.

Although drug budgets for most PCTs were increased by 10 per cent from the 2001/02 financial years to 2002/03, drug costs were expected to rise by 12 per cent. This represents an increase of over £670 million and even after the 10 per cent increase in budget the shortfall would be £110 million, or an average of £360,000 per PCT to be funded from other budgets.[3] These cost pressures are predicted to continue over the next few years and it is therefore very important that spending is properly targeted and waste avoided.

The Prescribing Support Unit has calculated potential savings for each PCT by a reduction in prescribing of premium-priced preparations, drugs of limited clinical value and drugs often over-prescribed, e.g. antibiotics, oral non-steroidal anti-inflammatory drugs (NSAIDs) and ulcer-healing drugs. Potential savings can be used for implementation of NICE guidance, government NSFs and the new 2004 GMS contract.

Prescribing data from the Prescription Pricing Authority

Data on the quantity and cost of drugs prescribed is available from the Prescription Pricing Authority (PPA) in England in the form of Prescribing Analysis and Cost (PACT) reports.[4] These reports, available in paper and electronic versions, provide feedback on the drugs prescribed and help develop rational prescribing. Additional information is also available to nominated users within the PCT, to compare prescribing performance between different practices within the PCT.

The PACT Standard Report is a paper report sent to individual GPs quarterly, but is also available monthly on request from the PPA. Quarterly reports are available for quarters ending June, September, December and March. The report shows the prescribing costs (total net ingredient cost) for the practice, individual GP, trainee and nurse prescriber, as well as a PCT and national equivalent practice, showing the variance from the same quarter of the previous year. It is also possible to see whether practice costs are above or below those of the PCT or national equivalent. The PCT or national equivalent is based on actual figures for the PCT or England respectively, adjusted to create an imaginary practice with the same number of prescribing units (PUs) as the practice. For calculation of PUs all patients under 65 count as one PU and those over 65 as three units, reflecting the increased costs associated with prescribing for older people.

The Standard Report contains data comparing the practice with the PCT equivalent in the six therapeutic areas incurring greatest costs in England in the previous quarter. These include a comparison of costs, items and average cost, indicating changes from the previous year, as well as percentages of generic drugs and new drugs (less than three years post-launch) prescribed. Costs and items are compared for the 20 leading cost drugs in the practice and 40 most expensive BNF sections. Graphs demonstrate the total practice prescribing costs by BNF groups over the previous two years compared with the PCT equivalent.

Each PACT Standard Report has additional information on prescribing within a therapeutic area, showing national trends and information relating to the specific practice. Increasingly, information from PACT data is being used as part of the appraisal process in general practice. The PACT Catalogue, which can be requested from the PPA, contains full details of prescribing listed by individual drug, but it is a very time-consuming exercise to analyse the full data on a regular basis.

Prescribing Monitoring Documents (PMDs) are financial statements issued to GPs as well as PCTs and the Department of Health (DoH). PMDs provide financial information about prescribing against budgets and show the indicative prescribing budget for the current financial year, total monthly expenditure, cumulative expenditure (April to current month) and forecast out-turn based on national expenditure pattern.[4] The statements show the cost of prescribing and help prescribers manage their budget. Currently GPs receive paper PMD reports but, from April 2003, electronic reports were made available to 200 pilot GP practices.

Monitoring the safety and quality of medicines

Regulatory scrutiny does not end when a drug reaches the market. The Yellow Card spontaneous reporting scheme operated by the Committee on Safety of Medicines (CSM) and the Medicines Control Agency (MCA) allows voluntary reporting of suspected adverse drug reactions (ADRs) by doctors, dentists, coroners, pharmacists, nurses, midwives and health visitors.[5] The scheme was set up in 1964 following the thalidomide tragedy, which first alerted the medical profession to the fact that drugs taken during pregnancy could have serious effects on the unborn foetus. Since then over 400,000 reports of suspected ADRs have been submitted to the CSM/MCA. These reports provide valuable information on drug safety in normal clinical practice, increase knowledge about known ADRs and act as an early warning system for identification of previously unrecognised safety hazards.

The CSM/MCA would like health professionals to report all suspected ADRs to newer medicines and vaccines, as well as serious suspected reactions to established medicines and vaccines. Newer drugs are marked with an inverted black triangle ▼ in the BNF, MIMS, and manufacturers' Summary of Product Characteristics, Data Sheets and advertising material. Black triangle products are monitored for a minimum of two years to confirm the profile of risk versus benefit established during pre-marketing trials, with the black triangle remaining until the safety of the medicine is established. For established medicines and vaccines only serious reactions need be reported. Serious reactions include those that are fatal, life threatening, disabling, and incapacitating or necessitating hospital admission. These should be reported even if well recognised. In addition all congenital abnormalities should be reported.

Since October 2002 health professionals have been encouraged to use the electronic Yellow Card via the MCA website,[6] but reports can also be submitted via Yellow Card report forms obtained from the CSM or inside the back cover of the BNF. Following receipt of a Yellow Card report the CSM/MHRA sends out an acknowledgement letter and, if requested on the Yellow Card, a cumulative listing of all suspected adverse reactions associated with the use of that drug is also sent out.

Another method of monitoring the safety of medicines following launch is prescription-event monitoring (PEM) carried out by the Drug Safety Research Unit (DSRU), based in Southampton. The DSRU is an independent registered charity associated with the University of Portsmouth, independent of any government body, including the Medicines and Healthcare products Regulatory Agency (MHRA). The PEM scheme is concerned with pharmacovigilance and examines the safety of new drugs intended for general use in primary care. The DSRU receives information from the PPA in confidence about patients prescribed a particular drug and a questionnaire is sent to the GP enquiring about any adverse events since starting.[7,8] The forms are reviewed by a physician on receipt at the DSRU and any serious, possibly drug-related events are followed up immediately with the GP.[9]

PEM seems to offer several advantages over the spontaneous Yellow Card system. For example, healthcare professionals tend to respond to requests for information more readily than they will spontaneously report problems. The programme also allows researchers to examine specific patient groups, such as children and the elderly.[10] PEM can also be used to calculate incidence data, since it holds data on the number of patients exposed to a drug as well as the number of reports of events, unlike the Yellow Card scheme in which the number of patients exposed to the drug is unknown.[9] Naturally it is vital that responders reply to the DRSU and send in Yellow Cards where appropriate.

As part of its continuing research the DRSU has recently become involved in a five-year research programme funded by the British Heart Foundation, to investigate potentially fatal cardiac arrhythmias associated with over-the-counter preparations for hay fever or indigestion. Consultant physicians and GPs are being asked to identify patients who have developed abnormalities of ECG or heart rhythm after taking medicines known to affect heart rhythm. Researchers will investigate a possible genetic predisposition and help identify those most at risk.[11]

Preventing ADRs

Some ADRs are unpredictable but there are nevertheless steps that can be taken to help prevent unwanted reactions to drug therapy. These are mainly common sense and include asking the patient about previous reactions to drug therapy and allergies before prescribing a medicine, and only prescribing it if there is a clear clinical indication, with regular monitoring to ensure continued need. Prescribers should only prescribe medicines with which they are familiar, preferably limiting their prescribing to a locally produced drug formulary. It is important also to remember that prescribers are entirely responsible for unlicensed medicines they prescribe and medicines used outside their product licence (see Chapter 10).

Certain groups of patients are more susceptible to ADRs and caution must be exercised when prescribing for patients who are very young, pregnant, elderly, or those with renal or hepatic impairment. It should go without saying that patients prescribed medicines such as methotrexate that may cause serious adverse reactions should be given as much information as possible about potential adverse effects so they seek medical advice when appropriate.

Reducing the risk of potential interactions

Swedish research has suggested that monitoring potential drug interactions might improve the quality of prescribing and dispensing.[12] A study of 962,013 dispensed prescriptions for two or more items identified potential drug interactions in 13.6 per cent prescriptions, with 1.4 per cent having potentially serious clinical consequences. Of the potentially serious interactions 2358 were between potassium supplements and potassium-sparing diuretics, and 644 were between warfarin and NSAIDs.

Prescribing software in primary care will highlight some but importantly not all potentially serious drug interactions. Also electronic systems are not usually used during domiciliary visits and prescribers must not become deskilled.

A recent study in Nottingham[13] showed that some potentially hazardous drug combinations are not detected by computer systems in community pharmacies. Prescribers should be aware of the potential interactions with drugs having a narrow therapeutic ratio (e.g. anticonvulsants) or those requiring intensive monitoring (e.g. anticoagulants). The possibility of potential drug interactions should be considered when therapeutic control appears to be lost in patients previously well controlled on drugs requiring regular monitoring. It is important to be aware that self-medication including herbal preparations (e.g. St John's Wort) and supplements (e.g. Co-enzyme Q10) can interact with regular medication. Even foodstuffs can affect certain medications. Grapefruit juice significantly increases the plasma concentrations of some calcium-channel blockers and recently the CSM issued a warning about a potential interaction between cranberry juice and warfarin.[14] Thus a careful drug history must be taken before prescribing. The BNF (Appendix 1) is a useful source of information on interactions.

Prescribing for specific patient groups

Certain groups of patients require more careful consideration before prescribing any medicines. These include: children, especially the very young; pregnant and lactating women; older people; and patients with renal or hepatic impairment. It may be necessary to adjust the dose or even choose a different medicine to treat these patients.

Prescribing in children

Doses for children are usually calculated on the basis of body weight or body surface area. The BNF gives some guidance for paediatric dosing but the book *Medicines for Children*[15] gives guidance on dosage for each medicine, licensed or unlicensed, likely to be prescribed in babies and children, as well as general guidance on therapeutics in children. This in the authors' opinion along with the BNF-C[16] are the definitive texts for prescribing in paediatrics. *Medicines for Children* unlike the BNF-C is not a standard issue and can be purchased by interested clinicians.

Some medicines commonly prescribed for adults should be avoided altogether in children. These include aspirin, which has been associated with Reye's Syndrome in children, tetracycline antibiotics, which interfere with development of teeth and bones, and quinolone antibiotics (e.g. ciprofloxacin), which can cause tendon damage.

Prescribing in pregnancy

The suitability of medicines in the pregnant woman depends on the stage of pregnancy. During the pre-embryonic phase, i.e. the undifferentiated blastocyst (which exists up to 17 days after conception), an 'all or nothing' effect is thought to apply. If there is extensive damage at this time due to drug therapy, failure of implantation and concomitant miscarriage can occur.[17] If damage to the undifferentiated blastocyst is minor and caused by an agent with a short half-life, the damaged cells will be replaced by extra division of the remaining cells that can then implant and develop normally. However, if pregnancy continues despite this damage during the pre-embryonic phase, the risk of foetal malformations is likely to be no greater than in the general population (one in forty). It is important to be accurate about dates (i.e. the last menstrual period) and there may still be a risk if the drug has a long half-life (see Chapter 2).

Developmental problems may result from second-trimester exposure also and drugs taken during the final trimester may cause problems during labour or symptoms in the neonate, e.g. delayed closure of the ductus arteriosus associated with NSAIDs or withdrawal symptoms associated with opiates, antidepressants, etc. Thus drug therapy in pregnancy must be continually reviewed to ensure a successful outcome to the pregnancy. The BNF (Appendix 4) gives useful information on drugs and pregnancy. It also includes contact details for the National Teratology Information Service (NTIS), which is funded by the DoH, to provide information on the safety of drugs during pregnancy, as well as pre-conception advice on drug exposure for men and women.

Prescribing in breast feeding

Many medicines are present in high concentrations in breast milk and may result in adverse symptoms in the neonate, especially in small or premature babies. It may be necessary to consider different therapy options for a mother who wishes to continue breast feeding or to temporarily stop breast feeding during the treatment course. A medicine taken throughout pregnancy will not necessarily be suitable if the mother wants to breast feed. It is important that a prescriber elicits the necessary breast feeding status of a mother. Appendix 5 of the BNF gives useful information, as does the specialist information service of the United Kingdom Medicines Information via its website.[18]

Prescribing in older people

There are many factors to be considered when prescribing for older people. Physiological changes associated with ageing may affect the pharmacokinetics of medicines prescribed. A reduction in liver size and hepatic blood flow may affect metabolism of some drugs and increase the risk of side effects. Glomerular filtration rate, renal tubular function and plasma flow tend to decrease with age, and doses of medicines primarily excreted via the kidneys may need to be adjusted, especially digoxin and other medicines with a narrow therapeutic index. There are also changes in volume of distribution with increased body fat resulting in an increased volume of distribution for lipid-soluble drugs, such as diazepam, and a reduction in body water resulting in reduced volume of distribution for water-soluble drugs, such as cimetidine and digoxin. The changes in volume of distribution are only clinically significant during acute drug dosing since at steady state the plasma concentration is determined by renal and hepatic clearance.

The response to medicines in older people may also be affected by changes in pharmacodynamics, with a reduction in homeostatic reserve and changes to specific receptor and target sites. Older people are more likely to develop hypotension associated with phenothiazines, tricyclic antidepressants, benzodiazepines, antihistamines and drugs used in Parkinson's disease. They are also more sensitive to warfarin and to the adverse effects associated with digoxin, but the mechanism is unclear. Benzodiazepines, especially those with a long half-life, can contribute to falls in older people, especially those whose balance and coordination is already impaired.

Over half of NHS prescriptions issued are for patients over the age of sixty[19] and between 5 and 17 per cent of hospital admissions in older people are thought to be caused by medicines-related problems. Appropriate prescribing and monitoring is especially important in older people.[20] Medicines-related problems are more likely to occur in patients prescribed four or more medicines, those taking warfarin, NSAIDs, diuretics or digoxin, and following recent discharge from hospital. Other contributing factors include confusion, disorientation, and poor vision, hearing or manual dexterity. Older people should be monitored regularly with a medication review at least every year, or every six months for those taking four or more medicines.

Prescribing in liver disease

Many drugs are metabolised by hepatic enzymes and hence require a healthy liver to be eliminated. Thus, patients with liver disease may show an altered response to medicines and prescribing should therefore be kept to a minimum. This is especially important in patients with severe liver disease in whom drug metabolism may be affected. The BNF (Appendix 2) provides information on drugs to be avoided or used with caution in liver disease.

Prescribing in renal disease

Drugs are either excreted in the urine or bile or metabolised in the liver and the metabolites excreted by the kidneys. Patients with renal impairment have a reduced glomerular filtration rate and this can lead to potential accumulation of a drug or its metabolites, depending on the degree of renal impairment unless the dose is adjusted. Appendix 3 of the BNF includes a table giving advice on the drugs to be avoided or used with caution in renal impairment.

Drugs requiring special monitoring

Recent research showed that 80 per cent of preventable hospital admissions were due to toxic serum concentrations of drugs, or abnormal laboratory findings, with inadequate monitoring seen in over two-thirds of drug-related hospital admissions.[21] This research shows us that prescribers must familiarise themselves with medicines that require careful monitoring to ensure they are used safely. Examples of these include warfarin, methotrexate and other disease-modifying antirheumatic drugs (DMARDs), NSAIDs, diuretics, lithium and some anticonvulsants.

Patients on warfarin therapy require regular monitoring of bleeding time by the International Normalised Ratio (INR) to ensure that they are not at risk of bleeding, or of developing thromboembolism. A study by the Cambridge Anticoagulant Service[22] identified the most common risk factors for over-anticoagulation as shown by an INR greater than 7. These included patients with prosthetic heart valves having a high target INR, recent antibiotic therapy, altered drug therapy or intercurrent illness. Fatalities have occurred due to poor warfarin control. In January 2003 the Chief Medical Officer wrote to all doctors about patient safety and medication errors due to poor handwriting following the death of a patient due to over-prescription of warfarin.[23]

Prescribers are responsible for ensuring that appropriate monitoring has taken place before prescribing warfarin and it is therefore recommended that practices have stringent protocols in place to ensure that appropriate monitoring is carried out and that the patient and all members of the practice healthcare team understand the procedure. Patients on warfarin therapy have an anticoagulant record book ('yellow book') with the indication for warfarin therapy, duration of therapy, target INR and details of INR results and warfarin dose determined by the anticoagulant clinic. Prescribers should check the yellow book before writing any warfarin prescriptions.

Methotrexate and other DMARDs have potentially life-threatening side effects and require regular monitoring by full blood count, tests for renal and hepatic function, and in some cases urine tests for proteinuria. Guidelines for monitoring should form part of a shared-care agreement between primary and secondary care so each player understands what is expected of them in terms of monitoring.

The National Patient Safety Agency (NPSA) identified 25 deaths and 26 cases of serious harm associated with oral methotrexate in a community setting in England between 1993 and 2002.[24] During that period more than 500,000 prescriptions were issued in primary care for oral methotrexate. Oral methotrexate used for treatment of severe rheumatoid arthritis or psoriasis should be taken once a week, yet the NPSA found that methotrexate was prescribed daily in more than 50 per cent of the 167 adverse events and deaths reported in patients taking methotrexate during 1993–2002. Although the NPSA is unable to estimate what proportion of the deaths or serious harm were related to human error it is important to be extra-careful when prescribing medicines such as methotrexate. The NPSA expressed the hope that GP practice computer prescribing systems can be adapted in an attempt to reduce human error when prescribing methotrexate, such as inadvertently hitting the 'daily' key on the computer.

NSAIDs are another group of widely used medicines with potentially serious side effects. There are recommendations from the CSM and NICE in an attempt to reduce potentially serious effects with these medicines. The CSM has issued advice on the gastrointestinal side effects of non-selective NSAIDs with recommendations to use those with lowest risk wherever possible, at the lowest recommended dose and not to prescribe more than one NSAID at a time.

NICE issued guidance on cyclo-oxygenase-II (Cox-2 selective inhibitors) in July 2001.[25] The guidance stated that these preparations should not be used routinely in patients with rheumatoid arthritis or osteoarthritis, but should be used in preference to standard NSAIDs only when clearly indicated in patients at 'high risk' of developing serious gastrointestinal adverse effects. These include patients over 65 years of age, those taking other medicines likely to contribute to gastrointestinal adverse effects, those with serious co-morbidity and those requiring long-term treatment with maximum doses of standard NSAIDs. Other medicines such as lithium require regular monitoring of plasma levels to prevent toxicity. Shared-care arrangements may be in place with secondary care for monitoring. This is featured as a clinical marker in the 2004 GMS contract.

Monitoring requirements for patients with chronic diseases

Medicines must be shown to be clinically effective as well as safe. It is estimated that up to half of all patients with chronic conditions (especially older people) do not take their medicines as intended.[26] It is not acceptable to prescribe an antihypertensive medicine for a patient with high blood pressure if the blood pressure is not regularly monitored to review efficacy of the prescribed medicine. Similarly patients on medication for diabetes, asthmatic patients requiring inhaler therapy and patients prescribed statins for high-serum cholesterol should be regularly reviewed. The most expensive treatment is one that doesn't work or get to target.

Compliance should form part of the regular review process. Patients using inhaler devices should have their inhaler technique checked regularly, to ensure that they are still compliant, and if necessary additional counselling can be given or an alternative device prescribed. Compliance with dosage schedules should also be checked regularly. Some patients may find it difficult to remember to take medicines three or four times a day and this will often be evident from the frequency of ordering repeat prescriptions. It may be possible to alter the prescription to a modified-release preparation with a longer duration of action, which can be taken once or twice a day or even changing to an alternative medicine with a simpler dosage schedule. Older people and those with complex medication regimes may find it easier to take all their medicines at the same time of day if possible to aid compliance. Monitored dosage systems are also available to help patients with compliance problems.

Patients with chronic diseases must be regularly followed up and reviewed to ensure that they receive optimal therapy. Review of medicines prescribed should form part of the regular review of these patients, in line with national guidelines such as NICE or those produced by the British Hypertension Society, British Hyperlipidaemia Association and the British Thoracic Society.

Audit

In order to investigate compliance in any particular prescribing situation we need to consider the use of medical audit. We can define medical audit as a formal look at the quality of practice in a particular area of medicine and involves benchmarking this against best practice.[27] The steps involved in undertaking such an audit include the following:

1. Defining the aims of the audit.
2. Researching the background to the area and clearly identifying the relevant issues.
3. Creation of an audit team, with clear identification of responsibilities. This targets appropriate tasks to the correct individual.
4. Clear definition of indicators, with an understanding of the reliability of the chosen measures.
5. Defining how the data will be collected and analysed.
6. A clear definition of the level that the chosen indicator should reach.

Audit therefore is looking at a form of compliance and, rather than just being considered a cycle (Figure 9.1), could be thought of as a helix, thus encouraging the concept of a continuing process.

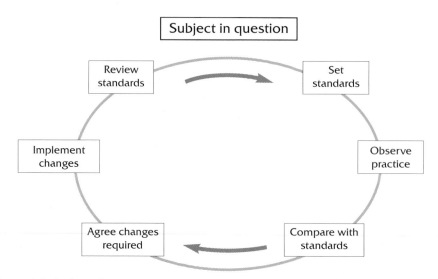

Figure 9.1: Audit cycle

Audit is being used for performance review in primary care at a massive level as part of the 2004 GMS contract. Furthermore, aspects of audit may well form part of the GP re-accreditation process in the future. Simple projects, e.g. aspirin and coronary heart disease (CHD), amiodarone and thyroid function tests (TFTs), thyroxine and TFTs, can be considered good examples of prescribing audit.

The results from computer searches needed to carry out audits can be only as good as the data held on the computer databases. Hence the saying 'Rubbish in, rubbish out'. To improve the quality of data, all members of a practice healthcare team need to standardise the way information is coded and recorded on the practice computer database. This requires the using of agreed 'Read Codes' to ensure that the information is clearly accessible. There are implications both clinically in relation to patient care as well as financially, since the GP contract and local Prescribing Incentive Schemes offer financial rewards for attaining certain targets, based on the results from practice audit.

The need for fast and efficient searching, and hence audit, has never been as necessary as it is now. As we look at the data collection required in the 2004 GP contract, it becomes all too clear that computer-held information is the only way forwards. Time and investment by primary care to collate the required information on computer databases is and will be time well spent.

Repeat prescribing

Repeat prescribing accounts for a frightening 70–80 per cent of the entire prescribing budget in primary care. A repeat prescribing system allows a patient stabilised on regular medication to obtain repeat prescriptions, without a consultation. The prescriber determines the interval between prescriptions (ideally no more than four weeks) as well as negotiating with the patient the number of repeat prescriptions to be issued before re-authorisation and hence review.

Repeat prescribing systems have many pitfalls including safety issues for medicines requiring regular monitoring as well as potential waste due to patients over-ordering or ordering medicines no longer required. Although various schemes have been introduced to help simplify the process, practices need to develop a repeat prescribing system to suit their own particular requirements and ensure that it is understood by patients and practice staff. The new GMS contract for GPs includes quality indicators relating to medicines management.[28] These relate to the time between ordering and receiving repeat prescriptions, and frequency of medication review. Clearly patient satisfaction is important. However, in the authors' opinion, quality is of prime importance.

Managing repeat prescribing can be time consuming for everyone involved. A good repeat prescribing system should be a partnership between the patient, the practice and the pharmacist. The system must ensure that the prescription generated is accurate. Ideally all medicines available as repeat prescriptions should be issued at the same time, for the same duration, to rationalise patient requests for repeat prescriptions. There should also be a mechanism to indicate over- or under-ordering repeat medicines to highlight potential compliance problems. In older patients or those on medicines requiring regular monitoring the re-authorisation of repeat prescriptions should link in with regular review and monitoring.

The practice must also develop procedures for recording changes to repeat prescriptions. If a dose is altered or a medicine discontinued the reason should be recorded in the patient's record, to ensure that all members of the practice healthcare team understand the reason for the change and that an incorrect prescription is not issued in error. It is also vital to have good communication between primary and secondary care, with a watertight system in place to ensure that any change made to a patient's medication following hospital admission or outpatient appointment is recorded in the patient's records and the repeat prescription record altered accordingly.

Medication review in older people

The NSF for Older People[20] highlights the aims of monitoring treatment in this group, including ensuring that the medicine is effective, appropriate and not responsible for any medicines-related problems. An in-depth review of prescribed and non-prescribed medicines should be targeted at older people at greatest risk of medicines-related problems. These include: those over 75 years of age; on four or more medicines; following discharge from hospital; in nursing or residential homes; with known medicines-related problems; or those with dizziness or confusion, which could be medicines-related.

The medication review should be designed to check a patient's understanding of their medicines, as well as monitoring requirements and any side effects experienced. It is also important to enquire about any problems ordering and receiving repeat prescriptions, reading labels, removing medicines from containers, swallowing tablets or capsules, or remembering to take the medicines.

Following the medication review it may be possible to rationalise prescribing and simplify the medication regime to improve patient safety and reduce potential waste.

With an expanding elderly population combined with an increasing number of prescribed drugs this may seem a daunting task. However, it is well recognised that this is an important area that needs increased vigilance.

Electronic prescribing

The NHS Plan and Information for Health outlined developments in information technology for general practice designed to revolutionise the way GPs relate to their patients.[29] One of these initiatives is that, following pilot schemes, patients will be able to access their electronic patient record and order repeat prescriptions electronically directly from the pharmacy. This will hopefully reduce waste due to patients over-ordering items or ordering items before they are required. The scheme relies upon good two-way communication between GP and community pharmacist to ensure that any changes to the medication are notified to the pharmacist, who in turn informs the GP of any potential problems. Concerns surrounding security and confidentiality have been raised by patients, GPs and community pharmacists in a survey of 200 GPs, 200 community pharmacists and 800 patients.[30]

Repeat dispensing schemes

The DoH highlighted the need for repeat dispensing schemes, whereby patients with chronic diseases obtain their repeat medicines for up to a year without having to contact their GP.[31] Thirty-two PCTs were involved with initial pathfinder sites to evaluate the scheme, with another 40 sites to be implemented early in 2004. The scheme has the potential to relieve pressure on GP practices by reducing requests for routine repeat prescriptions, as well as reducing waste due to over-ordering, and better utilising the skills of the community pharmacist in helping patients manage their medicines.[32]

Participation in the scheme is voluntary and patients need to understand that information about their medicines will be passed backwards and forwards between prescriber and pharmacist.

The prescriber's software system generates the repeatable prescription, as well as a series of 'batch issues' up to one year as chosen by the prescriber. In addition to the usual prescription requirements the repeatable prescription also specifies the number of issues and the dispensing interval (e.g. monthly, weekly, quarterly). The repeatable prescription is the legal prescription and must be signed by the prescriber and used each time a repeat issue is dispensed. The batch issues are for reimbursement use only and are not signed by the prescriber.

Currently all drugs that can be prescribed on the NHS are included in the repeat dispensing scheme except Schedule 2 and 3 Controlled Drugs, but these may be included in future following further discussion with the Home Office.

The scheme should improve communication between the GP and the pharmacist since the prescriber will need to inform the pharmacist of any change in medication. The pharmacist in turn will inform the prescriber about any medicines-related problems experienced by the patient. Although the scheme should result in a reduction in GP workload, some GPs may see this as further erosion of their traditional prescribing role.

There have also been concerns expressed that patients will be tied to one pharmacy, restricting their choice, but since the scheme is voluntary no patient has to participate if not prepared to use one pharmacy for the duration of the repeat dispensing prescription. In addition there is the potential for improved patient safety since the community pharmacist will have an accurate record of the medicines prescribed for the patient and will be better able to advise on the suitability of over-the-counter preparations.

The practice-based pharmacist

There have been pharmacists working within GP practices for over ten years. These practice-based pharmacists were initially involved in measures to reduce prescribing costs by analysis of practice prescribing patterns. A postal questionnaire sent to practice-based pharmacists in two NHS regions in the UK showed that the numbers with hospital and community background were similar, most had been registered for over 10 years and most worked in practices on a part-time basis only.[33] This diversity of background and experience allows practice-based pharmacists to perform differing roles within different practices.

Practice-based pharmacists have worked with practices to support and facilitate increased generic prescribing, switching to more cost-effective preparations and reducing waste.[34] The skills of practice-based pharmacists can also be utilised to perform medication review in older people. A randomised controlled trial comparing clinical medication review by a pharmacist against normal general practice review was carried out involving 1188 patients in the community, aged 65 or more, receiving at least one repeat prescription.[35] Review by a pharmacist resulted in more alterations to repeat prescriptions and lower prescribing costs compared with normal review, with no increase in use of healthcare services. Another randomised controlled study[36] involved 332 patients aged 65 and over, with at least two chronic disease states, regularly taking at least four prescribed medicines. Pharmacists successfully used information from the practice computer, medical records and patient interviews to identify and resolve pharmaceutical care issues.

Increased emphasis on medicines management, implementation of NICE guidance and the medication review targets set by the NSF for Older People[20] would be difficult to achieve without the input from practice-based pharmacists. In addition to medication review pharmacists can assist in medicines management provision, including management of repeat prescribing, medication monitoring, service to care homes and patient education.[26] The new GP contract and PCT prescribing incentive schemes include financial incentives for achieving targets in chronic disease management. Practices will look towards their practice-based pharmacists to help achieve savings to counteract the resultant increased expenditure on prescribing.

This chapter has considered various aspects about the need for the monitoring of prescribing. However, it is of importance both for our patients and for the prescribing practitioners from a medicolegal viewpoint also. It is to this latter issue that we now turn in the next chapter.

References

1. *Pharmacy in the Future – Implementing the NHS Plan. A Programme for Pharmacy in the National Health Service*. London: DoH, 2000.
2. *Audit Commission. A Spoonful of Sugar: Medicines Management in NHS Hospitals*. London: Audit Commission, 2001. www.audit-commission.gov.uk [accessed May 2006].
3. *Primary Care Prescribing. A Bulletin for Primary Care Trusts*. London: Audit Commission, 2003.
4. Prescription Pricing Authority. www.ppa.org.uk/ppa/Pct/pctReports.htm [accessed May 2006].
5. Medicines Control Agency. www.mca.gov.uk/ [accessed May 2006].
6. www.mhra.gov.uk/home/idcplg?IdcService=SS_GET_PAGE&nodeId=287 [accessed May 2006].
7. Rawson NS, Pearce GL and Inman WH. Prescription-event monitoring: methodology and recent progress. *J Clin Epidemiol* 1990; **43**: 509–22.
8. Andrew JE, Prescott P, Smith TM, *et al*. Testing for adverse reactions using prescription event monitoring. *Stat Med* 1996; **15**: 987–1002.
9. Drug Safety Research Unit. www.dsru.org/pem2002.html [accessed May 2006].
10. Mackay FJ. Post-marketing studies: The work of the Drug Safety Research Unit. *Drug Saf* 1998; **19**: 343–53.
11. Drug Safety Research Unit. www.dsru.org/news2002.html [accessed May 2006].
12. Merlo J, Liedholm H, Lindblad U, *et al*. Prescriptions with potential drug interactions dispensed at Swedish pharmacies in January 1999: Cross sectional study. *BMJ* 2001; **323**: 427–8.
13. Chen Y–F, Neil KE, Avery AJ, *et al*. Prescriptions with potentially hazardous/contraindicated drug combinations presented to community pharmacies. *Int J Pharm Pract* 2002: **10** (supplement): R29.
14. Possible interaction between warfarin and cranberry juice. *MCA/CSM Current Problems in Pharmacovigilance* 2003; **29**: 8.
15. Royal College of Paediatrics and Child Health/Neonatal and Paediatric Pharmacists Group. *Medicines for Children*. London: RCPCH Publications Limited, 2003.
16. www.bnfc.nhs.uk [accessed May 2006].
17. McElhatton P. General principles of drug use in pregnancy. *Pharm J* 2003; **270**: 232–4.
18. United Kingdom Medicines Information. www.UKMI.nhs.uk [accessed May 2006].
19. www.dh.gov.uk/PublicationsAndStatistics/Statistics/StatisticalWorkAreas/StatisticalHealth Care/StatisticalHealthCareArticle/fs/en?CONTENT_ID=4086488&chk=QcJvjQ [accessed May 2006].
20. *Medicines and Older People: Implementing Medicines-Related Aspects of the NSF for Older People*. London: DoH, 2001. www.dh.gov.uk/PolicyAndGuidance/HealthAndSocialCareTopics/OlderPeoplesServices/f s/en [accessed May 2006].
21. Editorial. Monitoring therapy. *Pharmacy in Practice* 2002; **12(9)**: 333.
22. Panneerselvam S, Baglin C, Lefort W, *et al*. Analysis of risk factors for over-anticoagulation in patients receiving long-term warfarin. *Br J Haematol* 1998; **103**: 422–4.
23. Communication to all doctors from Chief Medical Officer, January 2003. www.dh.gov.uk/assetRoot/04/06/54/58/04065458.pdf [accessed May 2006].
24. Mayor S. UK introduces measures to reduce errors with methotrexate. *BMJ* 2003; **327**: 70.
25. Cyclo-oxygenase (Cox) II selective inhibitors, celecoxib, rofecoxib, meloxicam and etodolac for osteoarthritis and rheumatoid arthritis. Technology Appraisal Guidance No. 27. London: National Institute for Clinical Excellence, 2001.
26. Medicines management services – why are they so important? *MeReC Bulletin* 2002; **12**: 21–3.

27. *National Service Framework for Coronary Heart Disease. NHS Modern Standards and Service Models.* London: DoH, 2000.
28. www.nhsconfed.org/gmscontract/ [accessed May 2006].
29. www.connectingforhealth.nhs.uk/eps/index.html [accessed May 2006].
30. Porteous T, Bond C, Robertson R, *et al.* Electronic transfer of prescription-related information: comparing views of patients, general practitioners and pharmacists. *Br J Gen Pract* 2003; **53**: 204–9.
31. *A Vision for Pharmacy in the New NHS.* London: DoH, 2003.
32. www.dh.gov.uk/PublicationsAndStatistics/Publications/PublicationsPolicyAndGuidance/PublicationsPolicyAndGuidanceArticle/fs/en?CONTENT_ID=4009188&chk=gPshGb [accessed May 2006].
33. Warner B and Goldstein R. *Pharmacists Working with Primary Care Groups, Who Are They and Where Do They Come from.* Health Services Research and Pharmacy Practice abstracts. 2001
34. Macgregor S. New challenges for primary care. *Primary Care Pharmacy* 2001; **2**: 2.
35. Zermansky AG, Petty DR, Raynor DK, *et al.* Random controlled trial of clinical medication review by a pharmacist of elderly patients receiving repeat prescriptions in general practice. *BMJ* 2001; **323**: 1340–3.
36. Krska J, Cromarty JA, Arris F, *et al.* Pharmacist-led medication review in patients over 65: A randomized, controlled trial in primary care. *Age and Ageing* 2001; **30**: 205–11.

Chapter 1

Medical jurisprudence and prescribing

Gerard Panting

Introduction

The only remedy the law provides to patients harmed through clinical negligence is financial compensation. Compensation figures are not just plucked out of the air but are carefully calculated. They are nothing to do with how bad the error leading to the claim may have been but everything to do with the harm suffered as a result of the error, and in financial terms what can be done to rectify the situation for the claimant.

Compensation payments comprise general damages for pain, suffering and loss of amenity, and special damages for specific losses including medical and other treatment, lost earnings, transport requirements, home adaptations with employment of carers to look after the patient and so on.

Calculating lump sum payments necessarily involves the grim task of assessing the patient's life expectancy as the overall award depends upon determining what is required on an annual basis multiplied by how long that money will be required.

For claimants and their advisers, the award of a one-off lump sum carries a number of uncertainties. Not only must life expectancy be assessed but also so must the cost of future care across that lifetime together with the likely investment return.

One method of dealing with the uncertainty over life expectancy is to make use of periodical payments through the purchase of an annuity. The Courts Act 2003 allows courts in England and Wales to impose periodical payments in place of lump sum awards, and the legislation also allows those payments to be varied upwards or downwards where there is a substantial change in the patient's condition.

The nature of negligence

To succeed in a clinical negligence claim the claimant must prove three things:

- first, that the doctor, hospital or other healthcare professional owed a duty of care to the patient
- second, that there was a breach of that duty
- third, that harm was suffered as a result.

Duty of care

The duty of care can be established in a number of different ways – sometimes without the doctor even seeing the patient. General practitioners owe a duty of care to their patients as defined within the GP contract but even casual advice to new acquaintances over the table at a dinner party could be sufficient to establish the duty. It is only where a doctor undertakes independent assessment on behalf of a third party, e.g. an insurance or employment medical, that it can be argued no duty of care towards the examinee exists but even here there is a duty to do no harm.[1]

Breach of duty

Assessing the standard of care provided by a doctor usually requires expert evidence. Since 1957, the Bolam Test[2] has been used to determine whether or not the standard of care is adequate.

Bolam's hips were broken during ECT. He alleged that providing a muscle relaxant would have prevented his fractures and to give ECT without one was negligent. When the case came to trial, experts for the claimant said that providing a muscle relaxant was mandatory and failure to do so was negligent. Experts for the hospital took a different view, leaving the judge with a choice between two contradictory and mutually exclusive expert opinions. Mr Justice McNair resolved the issue by stating 'a doctor is not negligent if acting in accordance with the practice accepted as proper by a responsible body of medical men skilled in that particular art even though a body of adverse opinion also exists amongst medical men'.

So, provided that the patient's management can be shown to be in accordance with accepted medical practice by reference to expert opinion, the doctor is, in theory at least, defensible.

A more recent case is often cited as adding a further gloss to the classic Bolam Test. In Bolitho v City and Hackney Health Authority,[3] the High Court held that the medical opinion relied upon must be deemed reasonable and responsible, and have a basis in logic. While some may argue that this makes the Bolam Test more robust, the counter-argument is that expert opinions have always had to withstand rigorous cross-examination and could only be relied upon to influence the court if they survived that test.

Delegation and responsibility

Delegation to medical staff in training or other doctors not themselves specialists in a particular field raises the question of how the Bolam Test should be interpreted in these circumstances. Is any experience a defence? Or, to put it another way, is it good enough to do your incompetent best? Or is there a minimum acceptable standard of care required, no matter who is responsible for delivering that care?

These questions were addressed in the Wilsher case[4] (in which a junior doctor catheterised the umbilical vein instead of the artery and failed to recognise the error). In addressing this issue, Glidwell LJ stated:

> the law requires the trainee or learner to be judged by the same standard as his more experienced colleagues. If it did not, inexperience would frequently be urged as a defence to an action of professional negligence.

> If this test appears unduly harsh in relation to the inexperience, I should add that in my view, the inexperienced doctor called on to exercise a specialist skill will, as part of that skill, seek the advice and help of his superiors when he does or may need it. If he does seek such help, he will often have satisfied the test.

Consequently, inexperience is not a defence in a clinical negligence claim. If care of a patient is undertaken, it must be delivered to a reasonable standard as judged by a responsible body of medical opinion competent in that particular field.

This throws a considerable onus upon general practitioners where there are shared-care arrangements. The GP who accepts responsibility for prescribing a drug with which he is unfamiliar must first learn what he needs to know about it, including indications, contraindications, potential side effects, monitoring requirements, adverse effects, etc. Simply to comply with a specialist request to prescribe a certain drug for a particular patient would not absolve the general practitioner of responsibility unless that same letter provided all necessary information and that, based upon that information, there was no reason not to act in the way that the general practitioner did.

Causation

It is not enough in a clinical negligence claim to demonstrate that the care provided was below par or that unexpected harm was suffered during the course of management. Compensation is only payable where the claimant is able to prove that harm resulted from a failure to provide an adequate standard of care or, in other words, compensation is only payable for harm that would have been avoided but for the doctor's negligence.

Although the causation aspects of a clinical negligence claim are often amongst the most difficult to determine, in prescribing cases causation is often straightforward.

Protocols and guidelines

Protocols and guidelines are now commonplace in virtually all areas of medical practice but no matter how well drafted they cannot legislate for all possible situations. Inevitably doctors will, from time to time, consider alternative management to be in their patients' best interests.

rsey Care NHS Trust,[5] the Court of Appeal had to consider the
ode of practice under the Mental Health Act should have. The code
for the guidance' of doctors and others (much the same wording as
reamble to many guidelines and protocols). The court concluded that
uld be observed unless there was a good reason for departing from it in
relat   in individual patient.

The same rationale should logically apply to clinical guidelines. Where, for any reason, a doctor decides to vary the management from the guidelines, he or she must be prepared to justify that variation by reference to a responsible body of medical opinion.

So failing to follow guidelines would not, in itself, be deemed negligent but it does put the onus upon the practitioner to justify his or her position by reference to the specific circumstances utilising an alternative, which in those circumstances is accordance with accepted medical practice.

Prescribing errors

In an analysis of 1000 consecutive clinical negligence claims against GPs,[6] prescribing errors accounted for a total of 193 cases (19.3 per cent of all claims), the largest category being failure to warn of or recognise drug side effects. In 3.6 per cent of these cases, incorrect or inappropriate medication was supplied to patients and, in 2.5 per cent, contraindicated medication was provided and, in a further 2.4 per cent, the wrong dose was prescribed. In relation to specific classes of drugs, the analysis revealed the following.

Steroids
Of all the alleged medication errors, by far the greatest number of claims (40) involved steroids – 17 oral (usually leading to osteoporosis and in a significant proportion this will collapse), 12 topical (six creams and six eye drops) and 11 injections of which six were related to Kenalog, causing subcutaneous fat atrophy.

Antibiotic therapy
Eight claims were linked to a previous allergy to penicillin and three to a known allergy to Septrin.

Phenothiazines
Ten claims linked to over-dosage of phenothiazines in the majority of which a degree of dystonia occurred.

Hormone replacement therapy (HRT)
There were a total of nine claims. Of particular note were three cases where unopposed oestrogen was supplied to women who still retained their uterus, in two of whom endometrial cancer developed.

Oral contraceptive pill (OCP)

Nine claims were related to the OCP. These included four, which involved the OCP supplied to epileptic women on drug therapy for their fits, usually Tegretol, where the antiepileptic caused induction of hepatic enzyme activity, reducing the effectiveness of the contraceptive. All these women were put or left on the 30 mcgs oestrogen pill instead of the recommended 50 mcgs version and unplanned pregnancy resulted. Another problem encountered with the OCP was thromboembolism.

Depo-Provera injections

Eight claims were linked to Depo-Provera injections.

Antiepileptic drugs

Seven miscellaneous claims were associated with antiepileptic drugs, not counting those four (see above) where interaction with antiepileptics resulted in unwanted pregnancies.

Addiction to opiates

There were six examples of cases where GPs had persisted in supplying opiates to patients who ultimately became addicted.

Prescribing for young children

The breakdown revealed that six cases involved drugs prescribed for young children, especially patients with diarrhoea and vomiting, which were not recommended at their age. They included such things as loperamide, metoclopramide, prochlorperazine, Kaolin et Morph, Zopiclone and Imipramine.

Lithium-related

Five claims were linked to prescriptions of lithium. Lithium is a potentially dangerous drug that can lead to hypothyroidism, renal or neurological damage, foetal abnormalities and sometimes death. Failure to check lithium levels and monitor aspects of blood biochemistry will inevitably lead the prescriber to an action in negligence should the patient come to harm.

Warfarin-related

It is perhaps surprising that only five claims related to anticoagulants but these are serious cases with displacement of protein-bound warfarin causing severe bleeding including intracerebral bleeds resulting in profound disability or death.

Non-steroidal anti-inflammatory drugs (NSAIDs)

Five cases involved NSAIDs and usually the adverse event was a gastrointestinal haemorrhage but in one of these the interaction was with warfarin, so it is included in the group above. As *In Safer Hands*[7] has recently pointed out, there has been a major increase in the number of patients receiving warfarin therapy over the past few years. Many of these patients are managed exclusively in primary care.

The paper sets out a ten-point checklist for practice systems to reduce the chance of adverse effects (see Box 10.1)

Mistakes with clomiphene

In sub-fertility treatments for women there were four examples of clomipramine being prescribed in error for clomiphene.

Poor contraceptive advice

There were four additional examples of this, not including the OCP or Depo-Provera, e.g. failure to warn when the OCP might be rendered ineffective.

Antimalarials

Four claims were linked to the prescribing of antimalarials. In two of these, weekly medication was taken daily in error.

Preventing prescribing problems

It is easy to see how the majority of these problems occurred and how relatively simple procedures might have prevented them.

One classic error is prescribing the wrong drug. Looking back through the Medical Protection Society (MPS) *Casebook* there are examples of chlorpropamide being prescribed or dispensed in place of chlorpromazine, Losec in place of lasix, and Noriday in place of Norimin resulting, respectively, in profound hypoglycaemia, acute left ventricular failure and pregnancy.

But before writing a prescription, the first thing to check is that there are no absolute or comparative contraindications. Simple things like not noticing the patient is known to be allergic to what is being prescribed, or that the patient is already on medication that will interact with the proposed treatment, occur recurrently. The commonest trap here is the multitude of drugs that interact with warfarin.

Next, it is important to check that the dose, instructions to the patient and route of administration are all correct. More than once melphalan has been given continuously, not in intermittent courses, resulting in bone marrow suppression and, in some cases, death.

Box 10.1: Ten point checklist for practice systems

1. Have up-to-date protocols for:
    - Initiating treatment
    - Dealing with high International Normalised Ratio (INRs)
    - Dealing with abnormal results out of hours
    - Dental surgery
    - Minor surgery
    - Co-prescribing and drug interaction
    - Transfer from secondary care
    - Discontinuing treatment.

    The end date should have been set at the start of the treatment. Before stopping, get written confirmation from the clinician who started the treatment.

2. Clear leadership and administrative arrangements
    - The clinician in charge of the services should be named in records
    - Any other staff involved should be named in records.

3. Education and training
    - If a GP has a lead role in INR services, this should be discussed in their appraisal
    - Record any dedicated training for practice nurses and administrative staff
    - Discuss possible warfarin complications with all staff as a significant event.

4. Have an external quality assurance process for near patient testing (NPT)
    - Arrange for this to be done every three months.

5. Routinely use Computer Decision Support System
    - Reduce the chance of transcription or handwriting errors
    - Use printed dosage instructions.

6. Put in place a system for non-attendees
    - On a weekly basis, identify those who haven't come for their INR check and follow them up.

7. Perform regular audits of the INR results
    - Use Rosendaal or Point Prevalence method.

8. Record any adverse events
    - Learning from thrombotic and haemorrhagic complications can improve practice processes.

9. Make sure all patients have a warfarin booklet

10. Co-prescribe by computer
    - Minimises the chances of prescribing drugs that interact with each other.

It is also important to ensure that the patient understands what side effects to report and the importance of monitoring requirements.

Patients must also be aware of the drugs they are taking so they can inform other doctors they may see in an emergency. And as a 'belt and braces' exercise, doctors must also ensure they communicate effectively with each other. The melphalan examples quoted above generally stem from ambiguous hospital correspondence.

Special care is needed when prescribing, preparing and administering drugs to children (see Box 10.2). Drugs that are relatively innocuous in adults may have adverse effects in children. Variations in height, weight and body mass can make them more susceptible; or they may quickly accumulate toxic levels as a result of slower metabolism and excretion. In many cases referred to MPS, errors occurred because the doctor failed to check the appropriateness of the drug and its route of administration in children or infants, or to prescribe the correct dose.

Repeat prescriptions provide a range of opportunities for things to go wrong. Unless time is taken to check that the requested drug is the one that the patient has been taking, that it is still indicated, that the necessary monitoring has taken place and that no new drugs have been prescribed which may interact with the repeated medication, errors inevitably occur with potentially catastrophic consequences for the patient.

A patient who was thought to have suffered a fit contacted his GP who prescribed antiepileptic medication and referred him for further neurological assessment. Tests subsequently revealed that the patient was not epileptic and the consultant wrote to his GP informing him of this. The letter was received by the practice and added to the patient's file but not acted upon. The patient continued to request repeat prescriptions for medication he did not require, which were issued without query. Over a period of years, he suffered side effects as a result of the medication and believing that he was an epileptic did not drive. When the true position came to light he sued his GP.

Failure to undertake necessary monitoring is another common problem. This may be due to lack of patient compliance, a breakdown in communication in shared-care cases or a failure to appreciate the existence of monitoring requirements.

Consent

There are a number of myths associated with consent law – perhaps the first being that consent is only required where a procedure of some sort is contemplated. That is not true. Any touching of the patient or provision of treatment requires consent. The majority of consent claims allege failure to warn or failure to inform, particularly relevant in prescribing when it comes to potential side effects and adverse reactions.

Valid consent requires competence, information and voluntariness.

Box 10.2: Advice for safer paediatric prescribing

- Limit the drugs you use to a well-tried few and familiarise yourself with their dosages, indications, contraindications, interactions and side effects.

- Refer to a paediatric formulary when appropriate.

- When writing a prescription include the child's age and write the exact dose in weight and (if liquid) volume required for administration.

- Always calculate doses on paper and get a competent colleague to check your arithmetic.

- When writing prescriptions, take special care in placing the decimal point and putting a zero in front of it.

- Never abbreviate micrograms.

- For amounts less than 1 milligram, prescribe in micrograms to avoid confusion over the placing of decimal points.

When prescribing for a child, it is particularly important to give the parents all relevant information such as:

- The name of the drug

- The reason for the prescription

- How to administer the drug safely (if appropriate)

- Common side effects

- How to recognise adverse reactions.

Parents must always be warned about side effects, particularly those that will be distressing to the child. It is also helpful to remind them of the importance of storing drugs in their labeled containers and well out of children's sight and reach.

Competence turns on being able to understand information about the proposed investigation and treatment, believing it and being able to weigh it in the balance to arrive at a choice. Consequently, competence is not an all-or-nothing phenomenon – the same individual may be competent to consent to one treatment but not another. Equally, competence is not about conforming to the norm. Competent individuals are entitled to make irrational choices (if they so choose).

Without sufficient information, it is impossible for anyone to make a choice. The General Medical Council (GMC) booklet on consent[8] and the Department of Health guidance[9] sets the doctrine of informed consent as the required standard for doctors in the United Kingdom. The amount of information that doctors should give to each patient will vary according to the nature of the condition, the complexity of the treatment, the risks associated with the procedure and the patient's own wishes. However, the acid test of required disclosure is all the information that is material to the patient's decision.

Unless consent to treatment is given freely, it is no consent at all. Any force or coercion clearly invalidates consent but many other more subtle factors may raise questions over the validity of consent. Patients who are pressurised into accepting a suggested treatment may claim that a metaphorical gun was held to their head.

Obtaining informed consent from adults

The GMC's guidance on obtaining consent sets out the information, which patients ought to know before being asked to consent to treatment or an investigation. That information is set out in Box 10.3.

If it is not possible to obtain informed consent from an adult in England, Wales or Northern Ireland because they are temporarily or permanently incompetent, treatment should be given according to their best interests as determined by a responsible body of medical opinion.[10] If, however, the incapacity is temporary, medical treatment should be confined to what is immediately necessary to save life or avoid significant deterioration in the patient's condition. The only caveat here is that doctors are required to respect the terms of any valid advance directive about medical treatment. Such statements are normally refusals of treatment, the most obvious example being that of a Jehovah's Witness who refuses to accept a blood transfusion. Such a refusal remains in force should the patient then become incompetent, provided that there are no reasons to believe that the patient was incompetent at the time the directive was made, has not changed his or her mind in the interim and that it applies specifically to the patient's current condition.

In Scotland, the situation is different. The Adults with Incapacity (Scotland) Act 2000 provides for the appointment of proxy decision makers who can make treatment decisions on the incompetent patient's behalf. Similar legislation is now contemplated throughout the United Kingdom but at the time of writing is not before parliament.

Obtaining informed consent from children

The test of capacity applies just as much to children as it does to adults. Although there is a legal threshold set out in the Family Law Reform Act 1969, which states that children aged 16 years and over may give consent to medical treatment, subsequent case law[11] has held that children who are able to understand the implications of accepting or refusing treatment are themselves competent and may consent to treatment on their own behalf. However, as the new DoH guidance[9] makes clear, it is still good practice to encourage competent children to involve their parents in decision making, but it goes on to provide the following warning:

Where a competent child does ask you to keep their confidence, you must do so unless you can justify disclosure on the grounds that you have reasonable cause to suspect that a child is suffering or is likely to suffer significant harm. You should, however, seek to persuade them to involve their family unless you believe that it is not in their best interests to do so.

Box 10.3: The information that patients want or ought to know, before deciding whether to consent to treatment or an investigation

- Details of the diagnosis and prognosis, and the likely prognosis if the condition is left untreated.

- Uncertainties about the diagnosis including options for further investigation prior to treatment.

- Options for treatment or management of the condition, including the option not to treat.

- The purpose of a proposed investigation or treatment; details of the procedures or therapies involved, including subsidiary treatment such as methods of pain relief; how the patient should prepare for the procedure; and details of what the patient might experience during or after the procedure including common and serious side effects.

- For each option, explanations of the likely benefits and the probabilities of success; and discussion of any serious or frequently occurring risks, and of any lifestyle changes that may be caused by, or necessitated by, the treatment.

- Advice about whether a proposed treatment is experimental.

- How and when the patient's condition and any side effects will be monitored or re-assessed.

- The name of the doctor who will have overall responsibility for the treatment and, where appropriate, names of the senior members of his or her team.

- Whether doctors in training will be involved, and the extent to which students may be involved in an investigation or treatment.

- A reminder that patients can change their minds about a decision at any time.

- A reminder that patients have a right to seek a second opinion.

- Where applicable, details of costs or changes that the patient may have to meet.

Source: *Seeking Patients' Consent: The Ethical Considerations*. London: General Medical Council, November 1998.

Box 10.4: People with parental responsibility

The Children Act 1989 sets out who has parental responsibility and these include:

- The child's parents if married to each other at the time of conception or birth

- The child's mother, but not father if they were not so married *unless* the father has acquired parental responsibility via a court order or a parental responsibility agreement or the couple subsequently marry

- The child's legally appointed guardian – appointed either by a court or by a parent with parental responsibility in the event of their own death

- A person in whose favour a court has made a residence order concerning the child

- A local authority designated in a care order in respect of the child (but not where the child is being looked after under section 20 of the Children Act, also known as being 'accommodated' or in 'voluntary care')

- A local authority or other authorised person who holds an emergency protection order in respect of the child.

Source: *Seeking Consent: Working with Children*. London: DoH, November 2001.

If a child is not competent, consent should be sought from someone with parental responsibility. Box 10.4 sets out those included in this group.

A good, if perhaps over-rehearsed, example of how consent law applies to prescribing practice is the use of mefloquine for malaria prophylaxis. Many holiday-makers destined for locations where malaria is endemic will seek advice from their GP or travel clinic. But what should they be told about the potential adverse effects of this drug?

In the *British National Formulary*,[12] the following information is available:

Indications

Chemoprophylaxis of malaria, treatment of uncomplicated falciparum malaria and chloroquine-resistant vivax malaria.

Cautions

Exclude pregnancy before starting prophylaxis.

Avoid for chemoprophylaxis in severe hepatic impairment; cardiac conduction disorders; epilepsy (avoid for prophylaxis); not recommended in infants under 3 months (5 kg); halofantrine must not be given with or after mefloquine (danger of fatal arrhythmias).

Driving

Dizziness or a disturbed sense of balance may affect performance of skilled tasks (e.g. driving). Effects may persist for up to 3 weeks.

Contraindications

Chemoprophylaxis in first trimester of pregnancy (teratogenic in animals, manufacturer advises *avoid* pregnancy *during* and for *three months after*), breast feeding and history of neuropsychiatric disorders, including depression or convulsions, hypersensitivity to quinine.

Side effects

Nausea, vomiting, diarrhoea, abdominal pain, dizziness, loss of balance, headache, sleep disorders (insomnia, drowsiness, abnormal dreams), also neuropsychiatric reactions (including sensory and motor neuropathies, tremor, ataxia, anxiety, depression, panic attacks, agitation, hallucinations, overt psychosis, convulsions), tinnitus and vestibular disorders, visual disturbances.

Counselling

Warn travellers about *importance* of avoiding mosquito bites, *importance* of taking prophylaxis regularly, and *importance* of immediate visit to doctor if ill within one year and *especially* within three months of return.

Is it necessary to provide all this information? Would doing so deter a patient from taking prophylaxis? In the circumstances, might it be better to adopt a softly-softly approach?

Given that patients could choose holiday destinations where malaria prophylaxis would not be required, exposure to any of these risks is unnecessary (although it is acknowledged that many will have booked their holiday and may well have paid in full before taking advice). Nevertheless, travellers are hardly in a position to decide on mefloquine prophylaxis rather than alternatives unless fully appraised of all potential adverse effects. Prescribing without providing this information, no matter how good the intention, leaves the doctor open to criticism and possible findings of negligence.

Information leaflets

Information leaflets can be extremely valuable in providing patients with relevant facts in permanent form that they can refer to whenever they like. However, information leaflets should be seen as an adjunct to, not a substitute for, one-to-one counselling of patients.

These information leaflets also have considerable evidential value if, when explaining what information will be given to a patient, a defendant doctor is able to produce a dated leaflet setting out exactly what would have been said to a patient at that particular time.

The anatomy of a negligence claim

Since 1999 and the introduction of the Woolf reforms, clinical negligence claims in England and Wales have differed markedly from claims pursued in Scotland or Northern Ireland.

In England and Wales, the majority of claims are now dealt with under the pre-action protocol, which, as the name implies, precedes formal legal proceedings. The protocol is designed to ensure both sides have all the information they require to investigate the claim thoroughly, placing commitments on both claimants and defendants to cooperate in this process.

Once the claimant has obtained all the necessary facts to assess the merits of the claim, he or she must draw up a detailed letter of claim should they wish to proceed. The defendants then have three months to provide an equally detailed response. Either party is at risk of financial penalties in subsequent litigation if they fail to abide by the protocol. Box 10.5 shows how the protocol works in practice.

Many claims are resolved using the pre-action protocol, but if this is not possible the claimant may then decide to issue formal legal proceedings.

Formal legal proceedings begin with the issuing of a claim form from the County Court or High Court (for claims valued at more than £50,000). Full particulars of the claim must also be served setting out the allegations of negligence together with a medical report verifying the injuries claimed and a schedule of damages detailing the losses suffered by the claimant.

Once the Particulars of Claim have been served, the defendant has only 28 days in which to reply or face the prospect of losing the claim by default. It is not enough simply to deny the allegations of negligence – the defence must state which of the allegations are admitted and which are denied, whether the injuries sustained are agreed and the losses agreed or disputed. A Statement of Truth then verifies the document.

It is not up to the parties – the claimant and defendant – to manage the claim. That is now a job for the court, which will set out a timetable for all the procedural steps in the case including inspection of documents, the exchange of witness statements, expert advice and anything else that is necessary to prepare the case for trial. Failure to comply with the timetable may result in subsequent costs penalties.

The ethos of the civil justice system is one of openness so the parties are required to disclose all documents relevant to their own case even if it tends to undermine it. Both the claimant and defendant have a duty to search for documents, list them and serve that list on the other party.

The court will also specify a date when the parties must exchange witness statements, setting out the facts of the case as those involved remember them and the expert evidence that the two sides will rely on.

Box 10.5: The pre-action protocol

The protocol sets out commitment for both healthcare providers and patients. Healthcare providers are expected to:

- Ensure that key staff are appropriately trained in dealing with complaints and claims

- Develop clinical governance

- Establish adverse-outcome reporting systems

- Use the results of adverse incidents and complaints to rectify faults and improve services

- Provide clear and comprehensible information to patients

- Establish efficient and effective systems for recording and storing patient records for a minimum of 8* years in the case of adults, and 25 years in relation to obstetric and paediatric notes

- Advise patients of adverse outcomes, provide them with an explanation and, where appropriate, an apology.

Patients are expected to:

- Report any concerns and dissatisfaction to the healthcare provider as soon as possible

- Consider the various options available (the complaints procedure, alternative dispute resolution) in addition to litigation

- Inform the healthcare provider when the matter has been resolved.

* MPS recommends retaining records for 10 years after completion of treatment.

In the run-up to trial, the legal teams will review their respective cases in detail and finalise the evidence that they wish to put before the court.

At trial, the claimant must prove his or her case by adducing evidence. The case is opened by the claimant's barrister introducing the main elements of the claim and explaining on what basis compensation should be paid before calling the claimant's witnesses of fact to give evidence. Under the new rules, a witness's evidence is given in advance in the form of a witness statement so once in the witness box all that will be required is confirmation of a few basic details like name, address, etc. The vast majority of a witness's time in giving evidence is devoted to cross-examination by the other side and a short period of re-examination, which provides the home side with an opportunity to clarify any points raised during cross-examination.

At the conclusion of the claimant's case, the spotlight turns to the defence with evidence being called from witnesses of fact and experts. Once all the evidence has been heard, the defence and claimant's barristers make closing speeches, highlighting the main points of their respective cases.

There are no juries in clinical negligence cases in England or Wales, cases being heard by a judge alone. Although the judge may give an immediate determination, it is more common for judgment to be reserved, requiring the parties and their lawyers to reconvene some weeks or months later to learn the outcome and who has won.

Costs

Clinical negligence claims are notoriously costly, and throughout the United Kingdom the losing party in litigation pays the costs of the winner, which, in a complex case tested at trial, can easily amount to £100,000 or more.

Box 10.6: When writing prescriptions

- Be sure that the treatment is indicated.

- Check that the intended drug is not contraindicated and that the patient does not have a history of adverse reactions to it. Ensure that it will not interact with the patient's other medication and warn the patient about any potential interactions with over-the-counter medicines.

- Write legibly, taking special care if the drug name could easily be confused with another – use capital letters and give the generic rather than trade name.

- If you are not sure which of two similar sounding drugs you should be prescribing, check the spelling in a national formulary.

- Write clear and unambiguous instructions for dosage, frequency and route of administration.

- Note the prescription and any other relevant information (e.g. warnings given to the patient) in the medical record.

- Ensure that the patient is aware of what is being prescribed, and why.

References

1. Kapfunde v Abbey National plc and another [1998] 46 BMLR 176.
2. Bolam v Friern Hospital Management Committee [1957] 2 All ER 118, [1957] 1 WLR 582.
3. Bolitho (administratix of the estate of Bolitho (deceased)) v City and Hackney Health Authority [1997] 4 All ER 771.
4. Wilsher v Essex Area Health Authority [1988] 1 All ER 871.
5. R (on the application of Munjaz) v Mersey Care NHS Trust, R (on the application of S) v Airedale NHS Trust [2003] EWCA Civ 1036, (2003) 74 BMLR 178, [2003] 3 WLR 1505.
6. Silk N. What went wrong in 1,000 negligence claims. *Healthcare Risk Report* 2000; **7(1)**: 13–15 and **7(3)**: 14–16.
7. *In Safer Hands*. London: Royal College of General Practitioners, 2004.
8. *Seeking Patients' Consent: The Ethical Considerations*. London: General Medical Council, 1998.
9. *Good Practice in Consent Implementation Guide*. London: DoH, November 2001.
10. Re F. (Mental Patient: Sterilisation) [1990] 2 A.C. 1.
11. Gillick v West Norfolk and Wisbech AHA [1985], 3 ALL ER 402.
12. *British National Formulary*. September 2003. www.bnf.org/bnf/ [accessed May 2006].

Continuing education and prescribing

Tony Avery

Introduction

High-quality prescribing is an essential element of effective primary care, and yet it is not a topic that receives a lot of attention in medical undergraduate studies or vocational training schemes. Training for non-medical prescribers is also available, but may be limited in scope and duration. For example, nurse prescribers in the UK need only to undertake an approved training course (lasting 26 days) and have 12 days of learning in practice with a medical supervisor.[1]

Therapeutics is a rapidly evolving field requiring a very large knowledge base. Given the vast range of medications that can be prescribed in primary care, with new drugs regularly coming on the market, it is likely that most professionals involved in prescribing in primary care need to pay attention to this topic through continuing education.

This chapter provides an outline of the concepts of continuing education and current approaches being taken for GPs and non-medical prescribers, focusing on the situation in the UK. The chapter then goes on to discuss likely learning needs for professionals in primary care and some of the learning opportunities that are available.

Concepts of continuing education

There have been major changes in training for healthcare professionals in recent years, and the concept of adult learning has come to the fore in postgraduate education. This concept implies that learners already have a reasonable grasp of the principles of their subject, but are likely to have learning needs in particular areas. Approaches that use adult learning acknowledge prior educational achievement and trust people to take responsibility for ongoing learning. Key elements include valuing professional development, reflection on practice and learning from experience, including situations where things have gone wrong.[2]

Adult learning requires a mature approach from those involved in postgraduate education. Instead of providing 'off the peg' learning materials, it is important to help the learner assess their needs and to find appropriate methods for addressing these needs. This does not mean that there is no value in educational packages, some of which are

Table 11.1: Effectiveness of different methods of continuing medical education

Most effective	Less effective	Least effective
Learning linked to clinical practice teaching	Audit	Lecture format
Interactive educational meetings	Feedback	Unsolicited printed materials (including guidelines)
Educational outreach	Local consensus processes	
Strategies involving multiple educational interventions	The influence of opinion leaders	

Source: Cantillon P. and Jones R. Does continuing medical education in general practice make a difference? *British Medical Journal* 1999; **318**: 1276–9.

mentioned later in this chapter, but it does mean that the selection of learning methods should come after the consideration of learning needs. In many cases this means that professionals will decide on a mix of methods, e.g. reading, audit, reflection and implementation of new knowledge, rather than simply going on a knowledge-based course.

Having said this, it should be recognised that people learn in different ways and that continuing (medical) education has been defined as 'any and all ways by which physicians learn and change'.[3] Table 11.1 highlights the finding of a systematic review of the effectiveness of different types of educational methods.[4] It can be seen that the more active methods of learning tend to be most effective.

Current approaches to continuing education for primary care professionals

While adult learning principles give a lot of responsibility to learners, most healthcare professionals work within regulatory frameworks that require some demonstration that learning has taken place.

Until recently, all that was expected of GPs in the UK was to provide evidence of completion of at least five days worth of educational activities each year. Many of these experiences were expert-led lectures, which were not based on adult learning principles.[4] In common with experiences in other countries, this has led to the question of whether educational programmes measure participation or outcomes.[5]

The current approach in UK general practice is now more firmly based on adult learning principles whereby GPs are encouraged to develop personal development plans and these are normally discussed at yearly appraisals that have recently been introduced. While it is still possible for GPs to fill their educational time by attending lectures there is now a much greater emphasis on assessment of learning needs and seeking ways to address those needs in the most effective fashion. These activities are backed up by the Royal College of General Practitioners (www.rcgp.org.uk) and other organisations such as the BMA (www.bmjlearning.com). The RCGP also has a role in accrediting educational courses.

Most other developed countries have formalised systems for encouraging continuing medical education for general practitioners/family physicians. In some cases, such as the USA, this is linked to a formal re-certification process that includes a cognitive examination. In other countries the emphasis is on doctors demonstrating that they have addressed their learning needs and are practising in a competent manner.

Other healthcare professionals have their own systems for continuing education. For example, from 2005 it will be mandatory for pharmacists in the UK to demonstrate involvement in continuing professional development.

Identifying learning needs

The vast majority of prescribers will have been introduced to the main concepts of pharmacology and therapeutics in their undergraduate or postgraduate training. For most, however, this knowledge needs to be supplemented with learning about how to prescribe safely and effectively in primary care while taking account of patient choices and costs.[5]

It is unlikely that anyone working in primary care will know all the relevant information about every drug that they might prescribe. Therefore, in addition to learning about individual drugs it is essential that prescribers develop the skills and attitudes required for safe and effective prescribing.

One approach that can be used to help prescribers assess their learning needs is to consider these in relation to the different aspects of the prescribing and medicines management process. Some questions that prescribers might ask themselves are shown in the box. It can be seen that while some of the questions are knowledge based, many relate to skills and attitudes. For example, it is probably more important to develop the skills to access and use relevant information at the point of prescribing than to try to learn all the cautions and contraindications relating to drugs in a rote manner. Also, given the problems of non-compliance it is essential that prescribers learn to communicate effectively with patients and take account of their ideas, concerns and expectations.

Another approach is to learn more about individual drugs whenever a learning need arises. These learning needs often arise in relation to new drugs or those that are not commonly used by the prescriber.

In addition, prescribers need to keep abreast of policy developments. An important example in the UK is the Shipman Inquiry. Harold Shipman, a former GP, was able to acquire the means for killing patients by stockpiling large quantities of controlled drugs by collecting prescriptions on behalf of patients and taking unused diamorphine from the homes of people that had died. The subsequent inquiry identified profound failures in the regulation of controlled drugs in the community in the UK[6] and the government has responded[7] by introducing a number of changes including restrictions on GPs' rights to prescribe controlled drugs outside normal clinical practice and improving the auditing of controlled drug use. Prescribers in the UK will need to be aware of these changes in order to practise within the new regulations.

Continuing education and prescribing: learning opportunities

There are many opportunities for undertaking continuing education in relation to prescribing.

At a very practical level, prescribers need to ensure that they have sufficient knowledge of the therapeutic options when making prescribing decisions. This can help to ensure that patients receive effective medications with minimal risk. It is both unprofessional and unethical to prescribe without sufficient knowledge, and this means that sometimes continuing education needs to be done 'on the job' during consultations.

Fortunately, there are plenty of sources of information that are easily available including the *British National Formulary* (www.bnf.org/bnf/), MIMS ('*Monthly Index of Medical Specialities*' – www.emims.net) online decision support such as PRODIGY (www.prodigy.nhs.uk), individual data sheets (http://emc.medicines.org.uk) or review publications such as the *Drug and Therapeutics Bulletin* (www.dtb.org.uk/idtb/) or the *MeReC Bulletin* (www.npc.co.uk/merec.htm). These sources of information can also be extremely helpful for continuing education outside consultations, especially where they relate to learning needs that the health professional has identified.

It can also be helpful for prescribers to receive electronic alerts regarding developments in prescribing. One of the most useful examples is Drug Info Zone (www.druginfozone.nhs.uk). This is part of the UK Medicines Information Services and was set up to provide medicines information to the NHS. Registration is easy and users can choose from a range of alerts, including updates from the UK Medicines and Healthcare products Regulatory Authority (MHRA) and new publications from the scientific literature in different therapeutic areas. The information provided is comprehensive and timely, and is likely to address the needs of most primary care prescribers, particularly in the UK. In addition, GPs may find it useful to access continuing medical education websites such as BMJ Learning (www.bmjlearning.com) and Doctors.net (www.doctors.net.uk). For example, a useful learning resource on the BMJ Learning website is an interactive case history on 'Avoiding drug errors in primary care'.

Regular updates on prescribing issues are available in scientific and professional journals. Readers will be familiar with the content of mainstream scientific journals such as the *British Medical Journal*, but there are others that focus more specifically on prescribing, medicines management and patient safety. Examples include the

British Journal of Clinical Pharmacology, Drug Safety, European Journal of Clinical Pharmacology, International Journal of Pharmacy Practice, Journal of Clinical Pharmacy and Therapeutics, Pharmaceutical Journal, Pharmacoepidemiology and Drug Safety and *Quality and Safety in Health Care.* Few prescribers in primary care will have time to access these journals on a regular basis. Thus a website such as Drug Info Zone (www.druginfozone.nhs.uk) can be useful by providing alerts to relevant publications that can then be looked at in more detail provided the user has access to a library or to electronic journals. A number of professional journals provide information on a range of therapeutic issues. An example from the UK is *Prescriber,* which is also available online (www.escriber.co.uk). In addition the weekly GP newspapers in the UK give regular updates on prescribing, including summaries of key publications from the scientific literature.

In the UK, most prescribers in primary care have the support of pharmaceutical advisers, many of whom work closely with primary healthcare teams. These advisers are able to access information on the prescribing patterns of individual general practices and can, therefore, offer tailor-made education input in relation to any issues that they have identified. Also, in some cases they can provide continuing education in relation to learning needs that healthcare professionals have identified.

The pharmaceutical industry provides continuing education for prescribers in primary care. This ranges from visits to prescribers with the aim of promoting individual drugs, to more generic education in relation to prescribing in specific therapeutic areas where the companies have an interest. Also, pharmaceutical companies often sponsor educational events at which expert speakers are invited.

For those prescribers wishing to take a more in-depth approach to addressing their learning needs there are quite a number of options available for advanced study. Table 11.2 shows some of the courses available in the UK. These tend to be offered at certificate, diploma or masters level, and require payment. However, the Drug Safety Research Unit at Southampton (www.dsru.org) offers some learning resources free of charge. These are accredited for continuing professional development (CPD) and include introductory and advanced modules on safety of medicines. Useful information is also available on the websites of the Department of Health (www.dh.gov.uk), the Medicines Partnership (www.concordance.org) and the National Prescribing Centre (www.npc.co.uk).

Many of the university-based courses shown in table 11.2 offer flexibility for busy healthcare professionals. For example, most have a distance learning component and some are very much oriented around the prescriber's learning needs. Several of the courses are modular, giving the student the option of completing each piece of work in their own time. Not all of the courses are assessed by formal examination, with many using project work and some using reflective portfolios/learning logs. Those institutions offering a master's degree course usually require students to undertake some original research and to produce a thesis.

Table 11.2: Postgraduate courses in the UK relevant to prescribers in primary care

Venue/course	Aberdeen – Diploma in Prescribing Sciences
Comments	Distance learning with residential periods
Contact details	www.rgu.ac.uk
	email: pharmdip@rgu.ac.uk Tel: ++44 (0)1224 262502
Venue/course	Birmingham – Diploma in Evidence-Based Pharmacotherapy
Comments	Distance learning
Contact details	www.aston.ac.uk/prospective-students/pg/pros/lhs/03ebp.jsp
	email: a.c.hunt@aston.ac.uk Tel: ++44 (0)121 359 3611
Venue/course	Cardiff – Diploma in Therapeutics
Comments	Distance learning with a residential weekend
Contact details	www.cardiff.ac.uk/medicine/pharmacology/Diplomas.htm
	email: Colmansb@cardiff.ac.uk Tel: ++44 (0)29 2070 4028
Venue/course	Keele – Postgraduate Prescribing Studies programme
Comments	Mainly distance learning. Short courses, certificate, diploma and masters are offered
Contact details	www.keele.ac.uk/depts/mm
	email: b.oakden@keele.ac.uk Tel: ++44 (0)1782 584207
Venue/course	Leeds – Prescribing Management in Primary Care
Comments	Flexible modular course for certificate and diploma with additional dissertation for masters
Contact details	http://tldynamic.leeds.ac.uk/pgprospectus
	email: l.needham@leeds.ac.uk Tel: ++44 (0)113 343 1350
Venue/course	Newcastle upon Tyne – Diploma in Therapeutics
Comments	Distance learning with 12 days of seminars in Newcastle
Contact details	www.ncl.ac.uk/postgraduate/taught/course/38
	email: anne.makepeace@ncl.ac.uk Tel: ++44 (0)191 260 6180
Venue/course	Southampton – online modules on the safety of medicines
Comments	Accredited for CPD, the modules can be undertaken free-of-charge
Contact details	www.dsru.org
	email: webmaster@dsru.org Tel: ++44 (0)23 8040 8600

Conclusions

Continuing education is vitally important for prescribers. This chapter has outlined some ways in which prescribers can identify and address their learning needs (Box 11.1). There are plenty of learning resources available, including this volume, to support more advanced study.

Box 11.1: Considering learning needs in relation to prescribing and medicines management

It is suggested that prescribers might ask themselves the following questions to identify potential learning needs.

Deciding whether to prescribe

- Do I know how to assess evidence on effectiveness and safety of medicines?

- Do I know how to balance risks and benefits when considering whether to prescribe?

- Do I have the skills needed to elicit patients' ideas, concerns and expectations about whether a prescription is needed?

Deciding what to prescribe

- Do I have sufficient knowledge of the relative safety, effectiveness and cost of drugs available for treating conditions commonly encountered in primary care?

- Do I have sufficient knowledge of patient factors that need to be taken into consideration when making prescribing decisions, e.g. age, gender, co-morbidity, potential drug interactions, allergies and potential problems with adherence?

- Am I aware of how best to use the resources available to me to help ensure safe and effective prescribing, e.g. clinical computer systems, books and expert advice?

- Do I take account of patients' views in making prescribing decisions?

Knowing how to prescribe

- Do I know the requirements for issuing a legally correct prescription that can be correctly interpreted by someone dispensing the drug?

- Do I know the legal requirements for prescribing controlled drugs?

- Do I know how to give adequate instructions on a prescription so that patients will know how the medicine is to be taken?

Maximising effectiveness and minimising risk in long-term prescribing

- Do I recognise the need to review patients on long-term medication?

- Am I able to justify the frequency with which I review patients on different types of medication?

- Do I have effective systems in place to ensure that patients are monitored at appropriate intervals, e.g. if blood tests are needed?

- Am I able to explore patients' views about the medicines they are taking and their feelings about continuing with them?

References

1. DoH. *Extending Independent Nurse Prescribing within the NHS in England.* 2nd ed. London: DoH, 2004 (also available on the web: www.dh.gov.uk/assetRoot/04/07/21/77/04072177.pdf [accessed May 2006]).
2. Hayes R. Vocational and postgraduate education. In Jones R, Britten N, Culpepper L, *et al.*, eds. *Oxford Textbook of Primary Care, volume 1.* Oxford: Oxford University Press, 2004, pp. 543–6.
3. Davis D and Evans MF. The professional development of the family physician: managing knowledge. In Jones R, Britten N, Culpepper L, *et al.*, eds. *Oxford Textbook of Primary Care, volume 1.* Oxford: Oxford University Press, 2004, pp. 547–52.
4. Cantillon P. and Jones R. Does continuing medical education in general practice make a difference? *British Medical Journal* 1999; **318**: 1276–9.
5. Barber N. What constitutes good prescribing? *BMJ* 1995; **310**: 923–5.
6. www.the-shipman-inquiry.org.uk/fourthreport.asp [accessed May 2006].
7. www.dh.gov.uk/assetRoot/04/09/79/06/04097906.pdf [accessed May 2006].

Index